NO MORE
ANTIBIOTICS

BOOK YOUR PLACE ON OUR WEBSITE AND MAKE THE READING CONNECTION!

We've created a customized website just for our very special readers, where you can get the inside scoop on everything that's going on with Zebra, Pinnacle and Kensington books.

When you come online, you'll have the exciting opportunity to:

- View covers of upcoming books
- Read sample chapters
- Learn about our future publishing schedule (listed by publication month *and author*)
- Find out when your favorite authors will be visiting a city near you
- Search for and order backlist books from our online catalog
- Check out author bios and background information
- Send e-mail to your favorite authors
- Meet the Kensington staff online
- Join us in weekly chats with authors, readers and other guests
- Get writing guidelines
- AND MUCH MORE!

**Visit our website at
http://www.kensingtonbooks.com**

NO MORE ANTIBIOTICS

PREVENTING AND TREATING EAR AND RESPIRATORY INFECTIONS
THE NATURAL WAY

DR. MARY ANN BLOCK

Kensington Books
Kensington Publishing Corp.
http://www.kensingtonbooks.com

This publication is designed to provide accurate and authoritative information with regard to the subject matter covered. The purchase of this publication does not create a doctor-patient relationship between the purchaser and the author, nor should the information contained in this book be considered specific medical advice with respect to a specific patient and/or a specific condition. In the event the purchaser desires to obtain specific medical advice or other information concerning a specific person, condition, or situation, the services of a competent professional should be sought.

The author and the publisher specifically disclaim any liability, loss, or risk, personal or otherwise, that is or may be incurred as a consequence, directly or indirectly, of the use and application of any of the information contained in this book.

KENSINGTON BOOKS are published by

Kensington Publishing Corp.
850 Third Avenue
New York, NY 10022

First Kensington Trade Paperback Printing: August, 1998
First Kensington Paperback Printing: January, 2000
10 9 8 7 6 5 4 3 2 1

Printed in the United States of America

This book is dedicated to my children,
Michelle and Randy

The cases in this book are real.
The names have been changed to protect
the subjects' identities.

Contents

Preface

I went to medical school out of self-defense. My daughter, Michelle, had a chronic illness that became extremely serious as a result of the drugs prescribed by her physicians. Frustrated and desperate, I had to take matters into my own hands, including becoming a doctor myself! Today, as a result of what I learned, she is a healthy, productive adult.

My experience as a mother, medical student, and physician has shaped my approach to medicine. I believe in looking for and treating the underlying causes of chronic problems—not just covering the symptoms with drugs. I think that covering symptoms with drugs can be nonproductive, and at times, even dangerous.

In my book *No More Ritalin*, I explained my medical approach and discussed how drugs used today to treat the behavioral symptoms of attention deficit hyperactivity disorder (ADHD) can be detrimental to our children. When doctors are quick to prescribe drugs for chronic problems, it can leave the child with the original problem unresolved and cause serious new problems as well.

This is where I think the current use of antibiotics for ear and respiratory infections is leading. Studies show that antibiotics are not only contraindicated for most ear and respiratory infections, but can actually make the problem worse. In addition, and with far-reaching consequences, overuse of antibiotics can leave us with resistant strains of bacteria that will ultimately make antibiotics useless.

PART I

Why I Treat Ear and Respiratory Infections without Antibiotics

Chapter 1

What's Wrong with the Current System

Cari's Story

Four-year-old Cari spent almost half her young life battling chronic ear infections. Her mother breastfed her for her first sixteen months. During that time, she never had a single ear infection. When breastfeeding stopped, however, the ear infections began. The ear infections recurred frequently over the next two years. Cari was on antibiotics during most of that time, taking many different antibiotics on many different occasions. Her pediatrician prescribed amoxicillin, Biaxin, and Suprax, but none of these seemed to clear up the infections for any length of time.

When the antibiotics failed to clear up or prevent future infections, her pediatrician referred her to an otolaryngologist, also known as an ear, nose, and throat specialist, or ENT. The ENT physician performed a test called a tympanogram, which showed that Cari had fluid in the middle ear, and then recommended that Cari undergo surgery to place tubes in her ears to drain the fluid. The doctor felt that if the fluid could be drained from Cari's ears, the bacteria or viruses would not be able to grow and continue to cause infections. Cari was scheduled for this surgery when her parents first heard about The Block Center, a medical center for chronic health problems in children and adults.

A Close Call

When I first saw Cari, she had been taking amoxicillin "preventatively" once daily for a month. She was scheduled to have surgery for ear tubes the very next week. Her parents were looking for options. They did not like giving Cari antibiotics so frequently either, but they did not know there was any other choice.

On their first visit to The Block Center, I taught Cari's parents The Block System for Treating Ear and Respiratory Infections, and they began using it immediately. The next week, when Cari was scheduled to have tubes surgically placed in her ears, the ENT physician did another tympanogram to measure the ear fluid. There was enough improvement in just one week for the physician to cancel the surgery.

In one month of using my treatment, the tympanogram results were almost normal. (*See* Figures 1a, 1b, and 1c. The graph of a normal tympanogram should fall within the box. A line which is flat and does not enter the box at all indicates that there is either fluid behind the eardrum or a hole in it.) Within two months, the tympanogram was completely normal. Cari had been off antibiotics for two months and had not contracted another ear infection, nor was any fluid present in her ears. One year later, her parents report that Cari remained completely well—no ear infections, no fluid, and no other illnesses.

I had the opportunity to speak to Cari's father recently. It had been over two and a half years since I had first seen Cari, and her father was delighted and relieved to report that she had not been sick since. Her father said that now, when anyone in the family looked as if they are coming down with a respiratory infection, they start the protocol

Figure 1a

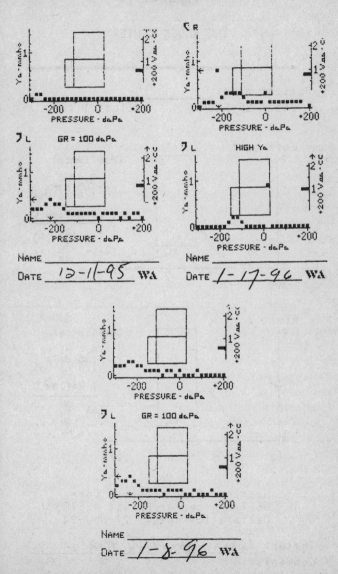

Figure 1b

THE BLOCK CENTER

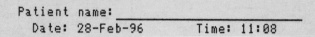

Patient name: _____
   Date: 28-Feb-96   Time: 11:08

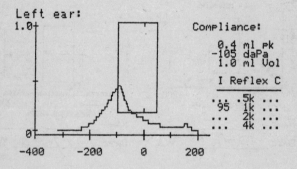

Left ear:

Compliance:

0.4 ml pk
-105 daPa
1.0 ml Vol

I Reflex C

95 · 5k ···
··· 1k ···
··· 2k ···
··· 4k ···

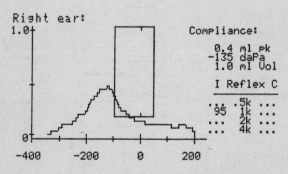

Right ear:

Compliance:

0.4 ml pk
-135 daPa
1.0 ml Vol

I Reflex C

95 · 5k ···
··· 1k ···
··· 2k ···
··· 4k ···

American Electromedics Corp.
AE-206 Tympanometer Serial #261850
Calibration date: 27-Nov-94

Tester: Terri Campbell, MA
Comments:

Figure 1c

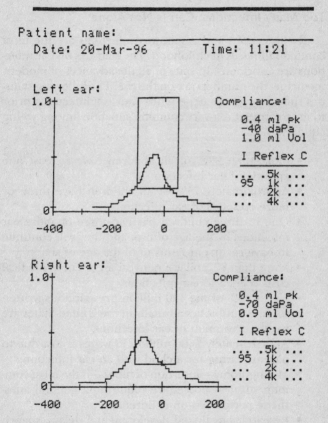

I recommended. They have been able to stop the progression of possible illness in all family members.

Too Many Infections: Cari Is Not Alone

Ear infections and respiratory infections are the most common illnesses in childhood. The statistics on ear infections are enormous. In spite of all the advances of modern medicine, the numbers are on the rise. The following statistics show that Cari's experience with ear infections prior to my treatment is a very common situation among young children:

- More than 90% of all children have at least one episode of ear infection.
- Approximately 75% of all children have three or more episodes of ear infections.
- One in three children has had three or more ear infections by the age of two, and they will continue to have recurrent bouts until the age of six.
- More than $2.5 billion per year are spent in medical costs related to ear infections.
- Up to 25% of the 120 million prescriptions written for oral antibiotics annually in the United States are for the treatment of ear infections.
- Approximately $600 million in wages is lost due to parents caring for a child with an ear infection.
- Myringotomy—insertion of tubes—is the most common surgical procedure requiring a general anesthetic performed on children.
- Research has linked developmental delays, speech problems, and behavioral problems to ear infections.[1]

According to research conducted by the Harvard Community Health Plan, ear infections account for one-third of all doctor's office visits for younger-age children.[2]

A Boston study of 877 children followed from birth showed 62% had an ear infection by their first birthday, and 83% experienced at least one ear infection by their third birthday. Forty-six percent of the three-year-olds had three or more episodes of ear infection.[3]

Additional evidence supports the theory that the number of children battling ear infections is increasing. In 1990, a U.S. government study documented 24.5 million doctor's office visits for ear infections, an increase of 150% over the number of visits in 1975. From 1977 to 1986, 42% of the prescriptions for antibiotics written for children under ten were for ear infections.[3]

Normal Is None!

Just because Cari's experience with ear infections is common among children does not mean it is normal. I remember one parent's response when I asked if her child had many ear infections. "Oh, just the normal amount," she responded. There is no normal amount of ear infections. "Normal" is none!

Ear infections are *not* normal. Just because your child has the "average" number of ear infections that does not mean it's normal. We used to think normal cholesterol was "250" because most of the public had a cholesterol level around that figure. It was the average cholesterol level found in people in the United States, but it was not a healthy cholesterol level. To put it in perspective, let me ask the question, "Do we want to be healthy or are we willing to settle for being within the norm? That is, do we want to accept the current standard, whether it is healthy or not?"

This was the question I asked myself twenty years ago when my daughter became seriously ill as a result of standard medical treatment still practiced today. My answer not only changed my approach to how I cared for my children, but ultimately sent me to medical school and changed the direction of my life. Before doctors made my daughter so ill, I was a young mother, not yet a physician, facing the problem of recurring ear infections in both my children.

I Have Been There, Too

I remember having only one ear infection when I was a child. I do not know if that was the "normal" childhood pattern then, but I do not remember my friends being sick with ear infections all the time either. I do know that I was not given antibiotics for my ear infection. It just got better on its own. Although it hurt while I had it, that was only for a couple of days. This was in the 1940s, and antibiotics were not so quickly prescribed.

However, both of my children had chronic ear infections, from the time they were just a few months old, and they were always given antibiotics. Their pediatrician was fairly conservative when it came to prescribing antibiotics, but that was the standard of the day.

My son's problem with recurring ear infections was more severe than his sister's. Randy's ear infections were so bad that we consented to have tubes placed in both of his ears by the time he was eighteen months old. While the number and frequency of ear infections were reduced after the tubes were inserted, he continued to have them.

Randy was on antibiotics for ear infections a good part of his first year and a half of life. It seemed that whenever he completed one round of antibiotics and was finally feeling better, the infection would return. Obviously, I wanted to spare my child the constant pain and isolation of being chronically ill, so I was willing to do whatever it took to help get him well. I certainly did not know there was any choice in the treatment he received. After all, those were the only two options his doctor offered: drugs and surgery. I did not know then, and did not discover until I went to medical school myself many years later, that drugs and surgery are generally all that doctors use because that is all they are taught.

Why I Went to Medical School

In my first book, *No More Ritalin,* I recount a frightening experience I had as a young mother. Physicians' overuse and abuse of drugs for chronic bladder infections made my daughter seriously ill—so ill I was forced to go to medical school to help cure her, which I did. What I learned there provided me with a stunning revelation of the problems within our medical system, and helped shape my natural approach to treating such chronic problems as ADHD and ear infections. In my practice, I look for and treat the underlying problem causing the symptoms, instead of using drugs to cover the symptoms.

In *No More Ritalin,* I explain, in depth, the problems in our medical training and how it affects the current approach to treating ADHD. The same problems exist in the treatment of ear infections. Physicians continue to prescribe drugs for ear infections even though studies show that children who are not given antibiotics recover faster than those who are. In addition, there is a disturbing consequence to the overuse of antibiotics—the emergence of stronger and more resistant strains of bacteria. To help curb this dangerous trend, physicians have been warned to prescribe antibiotics only for serious infections. So why do they continue to prescribe antibiotics for infections that are not life-threatening and can be handled by the body's own immune system? I found the answer in medical school.

What I Learned in Medical School

During my first year of medical school, I learned about the body and how it works. I took courses in physiology, anatomy, and biochemistry. I learned that our bodies are truly extraordinary. That first year helped me develop an even greater respect for how well our bodies function. But after the first year, my training was skewed to diagnosing diseases and prescribing drugs to treat the symptoms of the diesease. What could not be treated with drugs was generally treated with surgery.

The emphasis was on the disease process and how to treat that, rather than on looking for the underlying cause of the disease. We were not taught to look at what functional part of the body was in need of support. Even in this osteopathic medical school, the bulk of my formal training was drug-oriented, disease-based learning. I was very surprised to find this to be the case. I had specifically chosen to become an osteopathic physician because the osteopathic philosophy and approach are based on helping the body heal itself—looking for and treating the underlying causes of the symptoms. I believe that symptoms are clues, leading us to the problem. (I will discuss more about the osteopathic profession and its philosophy in Chapter 6.)

It's All About Drugs

Drugs are the staple of the American medical system. Drug companies are an important part of that system both philosophically and economically. Drug companies sponsor physicians' continuing education courses after medical school. The drug companies underwrite educational seminars and research studies. They send representatives to our offices, to take us to lunch and dinner. They give us samples and many clever promotional items, like prescription pads, office supplies, paper and pens, all stamped with their products' name, so we will remember them when we prescribe.

Even our medical journals are essentially funded by drug companies, whose advertising dollars support publishing costs. It should not surprise us to see that most of the articles and published research relate to drug therapy. Even double-blind studies, the gold standard for objectivity in medical research, are biased toward drugs. Double-blind means that two groups of patients participate in a study to determine the efficacy of a new drug. One group is given the drug and the other is given a placebo, an inactive substance, like a sugar pill. Neither the researchers nor the patients know which participants are getting which pill until the study is completed. Patients' responses are documented, and when the study is completed, researchers can see if there are significant patterns in the drug group as opposed to the placebo group.

This double-blind study method does not work for all treatments. It would be unethical to do double-blind studies on surgical procedures—that is, cut someone open and then not perform a procedure to see if they do as well as the patients who actually have the procedure. So our most trusted method of research relates almost exclusively to drugs. When there are new problems, we look for new drugs.

The standard medical approach to treating chronic health problems is to attack them with the same weapons, only stronger ones—stronger antibiotics, more advanced surgery. There is a saying I use often in my speaking engagements around the country which applies to the current treatment of ear infections—"If all you have is a hammer, then everything looks like a nail." If all you know is drugs and surgery, then everything you diagnose will be treated with drugs and surgery.

I believe that drugs are an important part of medicine. Drugs and surgery have not only improved the quality of our lives, but have saved lives. But as with everything, there is a point of diminishing returns. There is a point where overuse or inappropriate use diminishes the benefits. I believe that the current use of antibiotics for ear infections is just such an inappropriate use.

Chapter 2

The Problem with Antibiotics

Medicine Hasn't Always Been About Drugs

The practice of medicine has changed a great deal through the years, and there have been many different models practiced. It is important to understand them in order to understand how we got to the model we are currently using, the "drug" model.

Hippocrates, a Greek physician known as the Father of Medicine, founded what is referred to as the "ecological model" of medicine. Hippocrates was born in 460 B.C., at a time when the Greeks believed that sickness could be attributed to divine intervention. Hippocrates tried to find natural causes for sickness and health. He believed that the body had a natural tendency to heal itself, and if patients could heal themselves, they should take some responsibility for their health.[4] This philosophy was later adopted by Andrew Taylor Still when he founded the osteopathic profession. (See Chapter 6.)

In the Dark Ages, however, medicine followed a religious model. During this thousand-year period, people believed that disease resulted from our sins and healing came from certain religious activities. With the advent of the Renaissance, science broke away from the confines of the Church, and the door was opened to new scientific methods. In the 1600s, the microscope was invented, changing forever the approach to medicine. The microscope led to the establishment of the "specific etiology" model of medicine, which was based on the germ theory. The specific etiology model reasons that for any disease there is a specific etiology or cause, such as a bacteria or virus. In turn, a specific treatment, such as an antibiotic, kills the bacteria causing the disease. This "magic bullet" concept is still the dominant medical model today, particularly in the United States.

Since the discovery of antibiotics in the mid-1900s, the United States has very strongly supported the "specific etiology" model. It appears to me that the pharmaceutical companies who produce drugs, including antibiotics, exert enormous control and influence over the medical profession. So it should be no surprise that the primary treatment for ear infections is antibiotics.

What Did We Do Before Antibiotics?

Until the beginning of the use of antibiotics in the 1940s, there was no real treatment for ear infections in this country. Putting a hot water bottle on the ear and taking aspirin was about all that was available. (Other societies did have treatments, and I will discuss some of them in later chapters.) There also appeared to be fewer ear infections in children. A child who had one ear infection did not necessarily have chronic ear infections as we so often see today. As I have already pointed out, the statistics on the number of children who currently will have one or more ear infections, and the cost of medicating them and performing surgery, is so high it is startling.

What Is an Ear Infection?

I have looked into hundreds of ears and rarely seen a truly infected one. I believe ear infections are overdiagnosed and overtreated. Many doctors look into the ear canal and see a reddish or pink canal or tympanic membrane and diagnose an ear infection. However, if the child is screaming and crying or has a fever when the doctor tries to look, the ear will be red from the screaming and crying and the fever, not necessarily from an infection. Also, the inside of the ear will be red if the outside of the ear is red. It does not mean the child has an ear infection.

When you take your child to the doctor, the doctor has been taught to believe that you came for a prescription. I was told many different times during medical training that the patient wants a prescription when he visits a doctor's office, and if he doesn't get one, he will find another doctor who will prescribe one. Some doctors will diagnose an ear infection to justify giving you the prescription he believes you want.

In addition, many parents do not realize that antibiotics are effective only against *bacterial* infections. Just because you do not feel good, or have an infection, does not mean antibiotics are the solution. Most doctors are treating ear and respiratory infections with antibiotics without knowing if the patient has a bacterial infection that can even be treated with antibiotics. If the patient has a viral infection, antibiotics are useless.

Currently, there is no definite laboratory test to determine if a patient actually has an ear infection. In addition, no single therapy for ear infections is universally effective.[5]

The drug amoxicillin is considered to be the first-line drug for the treatment of ear infections. It is also very cost-effective. However, in many cases when the fluid is actually evaluated by puncturing the tympanic membrane, there are no bacteria present.

Puncturing the tympanic membrane is not routinely done, so we do not really know which, if any, bacteria is responsible for the symptoms. However, certain antibiotics are effective against most of the likely bacteria. This is why doctors just write a prescription for amoxicillin when they suspect a child has an ear infection. It's really just a guess, though. The doctor is "playing the odds." Some research indicates that amoxicillin may no longer be an effective "first-line" antibiotic for ear infections[6] because of bacterial resistance. If that is the case, the "bugs" have won another round against us.

What If It Really Is a Bacterial Infection?

I question the practice of prescribing powerful antibiotics across the board as the first-line treatment for ear and respiratory infections in children. Even if there is a bacterial infection, does the patient need an antibiotic treatment, or can the infection heal on its own, without the use of antibiotics? The answer may surprise you. *Studies show that 90% of all ear infections will heal on their own without medical treatment.*[7]

In the 1970s, a study in the United States measured the effectiveness of treating ear infections with antibiotics, by evaluating the records of children who were treated with and without antibiotics from 1950 to 1964. Interestingly enough, the group that had received antibiotics demonstrated slower healing, and had a significantly higher percentage of recurrences. When antibiotic treatment was started on the day the ear infection was diagnosed, the frequency of recurrence was almost three times that in the patients who did not use antibiotics at all.

This study clearly indicated that the sooner a child was given an antibiotic for an ear infection, the longer the infection would last and the more recurrences there would be.

Some might argue that inferior antibiotics were the cause of the study's findings, that antibiotic drugs were not as good twenty-five years ago as they are now. While it's true that the antibiotics of the 1950s and 1960s did not kill as broad a spectrum of bacteria as today's, I believe it is possible that our misuse and abuse of antibiotics is the real reason our children are having more infections today.

A more recent study showed that ear infections had a high rate of spontaneous resolution. More than 90% of the children studied were managed successfully without antibiotics. There was no increase in complications, either. The group that received antibiotics actually demonstrated slower healing and had a significantly higher percentage of recurrences, just as the 1970 study had shown.[8]

Adverse Reactions and Side Effects of Antibiotics

Every parent should know there are possible adverse effects from using antibiotics. All drugs have side effects, and the adverse side effects should always be weighed against the positive effects. Inappropriate and repeated use of antibiotics can adversely affect the immune system. Overuse of antibiotics can result in antibiotic-resistant bacteria. Some people develop sensitivities and allergies from repeated exposure to antibiotics. Another side effect of antibiotics is that they can change the makeup of your gastrointestinal (GI) tract. While the antibiotics are killing the bad bacteria that are causing you to be ill, they also kill the good bacteria in your GI tract. Without this good bacteria, you cannot break down foods properly, and digestion may be affected. *(See* Chapter 8.)

In addition, there has been evidence since 1985 that the insertion of tubes may lead to permanent structural damage of the tympanic membrane. It can lead to atrophy of the eardrum and hearing loss.

The "Just in Case" Theory

One mother took her child to the pediatrician because he had a low-grade fever and was acting fussy. The pediatrician could find nothing wrong after thoroughly examining the child—ears, throat, and nose all looked fine. The doctor even ordered blood tests, and the lab work came out completely normal. Then the pediatrician prescribed an antibiotic "just in case." Just in case of what? This is totally inappropriate. The child could have had a viral infection, not a bacterial infection, and an antibiotic will do nothing to help. This type of prescription writing has brought us to where we are today with antibiotic resistance.

This parent did not fill the prescription because she did not want to use antibiotics inappropriately. She also found a new pediatrician. In this case, since there was no apparent focus for the infection, there was no reason to prescribe antibiotics. This is just a shotgun approach. As physicians, we must be more specific in our diagnosis and recommendations. That is why I will do a throat culture before prescribing antibiotics for a sore throat. If the results of the throat culture show no signs of strep or other pathogenic bacteria, then I do not prescribe an antibiotic. Because a strep infection can have serious consequences, an antibiotic is appropriate. A throat culture should be done first to make sure strep is present. A physician cannot determine that a person has a strep infection simply by looking. Some of the worst-looking infections I have seen were not strep, and some of the mildest have actually been strep. A throat culture must be done to know the difference. In today's "managed care" environment, it is cheaper to give the patient a prescription for an antibiotic than to do a throat culture. However, cheaper medicine does not often equate with good medicine.

My approach in medicine involves trying to find the underlying cause of a health problem and fix that cause whenever possible. No matter what the problem is, using drugs usually means just treating the symptoms, not the underlying cause of those symptoms. If we can figure out what is underlying the ear and respiratory infections, we can usually treat it. Then the patient no longer needs to take the medications to control the symptoms, because they no longer have the symptoms.

In order to encourage a more conservative use of antibiotic therapy, it is important that we as physicians offer patients another treatment for infections, a treatment that will not place our health in jeopardy. This book contains such a treatment.

So Why Do Doctors Continue to Prescribe Antibiotics?

There are several reasons why doctors continue to prescribe antibiotics even though antibiotics are contraindicated for most respiratory and ear infections. As I explained, drugs are the mainstay of the medical profession. Doctors are trained to give drugs. Most of them do not know other treatments or modalities. So they keep doing what they know, even when research indicates otherwise.

Many physicians feel pressured to prescribe. After all, the public has been brainwashed to believe that drugs are the answers to all our ills too—the drug companies are now marketing directly to the public through television.

To test patients' attitudes about prescription drugs, in a 1997 trial, doctors followed one of three strategies for patients diagnosed with sore throats: (1) a ten-day course of antibiotics; (2) a delayed prescription (a ten-day cycle of antibiotics if symptoms did not clear up in three days); or (3) no prescription at all. Interestingly enough, the percentage of patients whose symptoms had resolved in three days did not differ significantly in the three groups, nor did their time away from work or school. However, the patients who were initially given antibiotics were more likely to *believe* the antibiotics were effective in treating a sore throat. Researchers concluded that although the use of antibiotics did not improve the outcome, it "medicalized" the illness by leading patients to believe that antibiotics are the best treatment for sore throat.[9]

But I have seen a different attitude from my patients. I find that if I take a little time to explain to my patients how the body works and to educate them on the limitations of antibiotics, they are then very happy to use drugs appropriately and do not want to get an antibiotic prescription every time they visit my office.

Some physicians fear that a conservative approach to prescribing antibiotics might indicate they are not "up-to-date" on the latest medical knowledge. In today's litigious society, some doctors fear indictment and lawsuits, and not being backed up by the medical board, if they do not succumb to their patients' wishes and prescribe antibiotics.[10]

Another reason doctors continue to prescribe antibiotics is because there is so much controversy in the medical journals on this subject.

Conflicts in the Medical Literature

One of the greatest difficulties for physicians in treating ear and respiratory infections is the massive amount of conflicting information in the medical literature. In 1987, a study was published in the *New England Journal of Medicine* on the effectiveness of amoxicillin. The researchers at Chicago's Hospital in Pittsburgh conducted a four-year study and found that children who took amoxicillin for ear infections were twice as likely to be cured as those who took a placebo.[11]

However, one of the Pittsburgh researchers disagreed with the conclusion of the study, and published an article in the *Journal of the American Medical Association (JAMA)* in 1991 citing no appreciable differences between the antibiotic and the placebo.[11]

Following these two conflicting reports, a family practitioner in Cleveland analyzed twenty-seven different studies on the effectiveness of several antibiotics to treat middle ear infections in children. But his findings, published in *JAMA* in 1993, showed mixed results. The study concluded that only one out of every nine children (11%) taking antibiotics for ear infections showed improvement. Of every six patients receiving antibiotics for fluid in the ears, only 17% improved.[11]

Other studies show similar conflicts. One study found that there was no difference in treating an ear infection with (a) the chronic use of antibiotics, (b) using tubes, or (c) just doing nothing.[5] Still another study indicated that 25% of all tube insertions may be inappropriate and that for only 30% were the benefits of tube insertion worth the risk.[11]

Even when the study results are clear, some doctors continue to recommend treating with antibiotics. Dr. S. Michael Marcy of the Department of Pediatrics at University of Southern California, Los Angeles, stated:

> Roughly one-half of patients will do fine with no treatment. Antibiotic efficacy is marginal—perhaps an extra 20% cured, compared with placebo. I'm not trying to say 'Don't treat.' But it doesn't make a whole lot of difference what you treat with, and the benefit that you generate is about one out of five children. . . . All drugs perform about the same, and placebo does almost as well as antibiotics. If you get about an 85% cure rate with placebo or drugs, the whole thing is about as good as chicken soup.[12]

Dr. Marcy went on to say that treatment is still appropriate because there is no way to know whether the child is one of those who will not do well without it. He went on to say that in a competitive medical environment, "sometimes you just have to give them the drug of the moment."[12]

I do not agree with Dr. Marcy's last two statements. Even if there are a small number of children who might benefit from the use of antibiotics, that is not a good reason to give antibiotics to everyone.

Even if I did not have another treatment option, which I do, I would recommend a "wait and see" attitude. Let each child's body try to heal the ear or respiratory infection on its own. Since 90% will do just that, the 10% who don't will reveal themselves soon enough. When they do, there will still be plenty of time to give them an antibiotic if it is needed. Remember, the studies indicated there were no side effects to waiting. With my treatment, there is no need to wait anyway. The parents can begin the treatment immediately. My experience has shown me that a larger number than 90% will respond and recover using my technique. This will leave a still smaller group that *might* benefit from antibiotics. If this new treatment is not completely successful, again, there is still plenty of time to prescribe antibiotics. We need to give the body a chance to do what it does best—be well.

How does a physician make a decision when there are so many differences in opinion in their own medical literature? How can patients trust that what the doctor is telling them is the best information available? In other countries, ear infections are rarely treated with antibiotics. Uncomfortable symptoms are treated with analgesics and the infections resolve on their *own* without complications. Why, in this country, do we continue to feel the need to medically intervene, even when it may be making matters worse?

The medical model is based on using drugs as the primary treatment for everything. When the doctor follows that model because that is what she has been taught to do, even when it doesn't make sense, what's the patient to do? Sometimes I think those practicing medicine forget to use common sense. Studies indicate that using an antibiotic will cause the infection to last longer and have more recurrences, and that using antibiotics will have serious, life-threatening consequences in the future owing to bacterial resistance. *Not* using the antibiotic will allow a cure in 90% of the cases, with no increase in side effects. Do you really need to be a rocket scientist to say that in these cases there should be *no more antibiotics!*

Although breaking the "antibiotic–ear infection cycle" will, in itself, be beneficial to the quality of your child's life, there is another, more important, reason we should let our bodies fight off bacterial infections. If we continue to use antibiotics indiscriminately, in the not so distant future we may not have any antibiotics left to fight new, more virulent and deadly infections, which claim more lives each year.

Antibiotic-Resistant Bacteria—The New Killers

If antibiotics are such wonder drugs, why are infectious diseases now the third leading cause of death in the United States? "Responding to a call from editors of the *Journal of the American Medical Association,* thirty-six medical journals in twenty-one countries published more than 200 articles on the growing threat of drug-resistant bacteria and viruses."

Some of the articles showed a connection between the overuse of antibiotics and the inability to treat certain diseases, such as bacterial pneumonia. Dr. Robert Daum, professor of pediatrics at Wyler Children's Hospital, said, "It is getting harder and harder to treat bacterial infections. The number of antibiotics is dwindling, and the bugs are becoming more and more resistant. We are going to be faced soon with infectious diseases that basically have no treatment options, like the preantibiotic era."[13]

Yet the overuse of antibiotics continues to expand. Most of our meats are from animals that have been fed antibiotics. We do not hesitate to give out antibiotics to our children for any little health problem, whether they need them or not, and often when the antibiotic won't even be effective.

It is important for doctors to consider this consequence when deciding to prescribe. Every time a drug is prescribed, it can potentially produce bacterial resistance. If the drug and the patient's immune system do not eradicate all of the organisms, the population of bacteria which survives will tend to be resistant. Once an organism begins to lose sensitivity to a drug, continued use of it increases resistance. Each new use applies the same selective pressures, but to populations that are weighted more and more heavily in favor of resistant strains. As a rule, broad-spectrum drugs induce resistance more often than narrow-spectrum ones.

> "The consequences of antibiotics have become clear," state the authors of "Wise Antibiotic Use in the Age of Drug Resistance." "Originally penicillin was reliably effective against the pneumococcus bacteria, the most common cause of bacterial middle ear infections. Today, however, about 40% of pneumococcal strains in parts of the US are resistant to penicillin. In addition, strains of other important pathogens are becoming increasingly resistant to commonly used antibiotics. Stepping up to more potent drugs is likely to make the problem with resistance much worse."[6]

Recent studies of outbreaks in day-care centers have shown that higher rates of infection with antibiotic-resistant bacteria correlate with greater previous exposure to antibiotics. The more antibiotics a child has had, the more likely he or she is to have problems with antibiotic-resistant bacteria.[6]

I recently attended a pharmaceutical company lecture

on bacterial resistance. I was excited, because I thought the speaker would discuss how we needed to be more responsible in light of current problems. I expected the speaker to tell us to stop prescribing so many antibiotics for so many problems which did not require antibiotic treatment. I thought he would impress upon us the importance of not using antibiotics unless they were absolutely necessary.

But this did not happen. The speaker gave an interesting talk about the history of antibiotics and bacterial resistance, and then proceeded to tell us which antibiotics not to use because they were no longer effective. There were no warnings about how abusing and misusing antibiotics had brought us to where we are today, or the danger that, in our lifetime, there really may be *no more antibiotics!*

I have also been disappointed in medical reports which continue to acknowledge the serious problem of antibiotic-resistant bacteria as it relates to ear infections, yet fall short of acknowledging the obvious conclusions. For example, one report states, "During the last 2 years, increases in penicillin-resistant pneumococci have been reported around the US. . . . Both the development of resistant strains and their rapid spread have likely been fostered and facilitated by selective pressure resulting from extensive use of antimicrobial drugs, the most common target of which in children, undoubtedly, is otitis media (ear infections). . . . Faced with the likelihood that antimicrobial treatment, particularly of otitis media, has been and remains an important contributor to the development of peumococcal drug resistance, I believe that we must curtail such treatment where we can do so without subjecting individual patients to undue risk."[14]

Unfortunately, the author goes on to say, "Antibiotic treatment should not be withheld because of the risk of side-effects, such as mastoiditis and other complications. . . . Overall, I believe that if the problem of recurrent ear infections is not seen as overwhelming, continued reliance on antimicrobial treatment of individual episodes is the best course to follow because this course appears to pose the fewest risks, and because acute otitis media recurrences tend to become less frequent and less severe as children grow older.''[14]

Even though this article recognizes that antibiotic use for ear infections is a major contributor to bacterial resistance, the author says to go ahead and use antibiotics indiscriminately anyway. Even though the author recognizes that misuse and abuse of antibiotic treatment of ear infections may be a major contributor to the bacterial resistance problem that we are experiencing today, he seems to be saying, ''Go ahead and keep prescribing antibiotics.''

Yet in countries such as the Netherlands, experts now advise prescribing only decongestants and analgesics at the beginning of the ear problem. They are not seeing any increase in side effects from this approach. In the United States, however, amoxicillin is typically begun at the time of diagnosis. If this fails, physicians are not in agreement as to what to do next.[6]

It continues to amaze me that the medical profession either chooses to ignore, or doesn't even realize, what is going on. I don't like to consider which is true. When asked why doctors continue to say there is not a problem, one prominent physician (who will remain nameless) responded by saying, ''They're either stupid or they're lying!'' I don't know which it is, but we have certainly had nearly fifty years to learn our lesson, and no one seems to have learned it yet.

Ear Infections and Antibiotic-Resistant Bacteria

So what part does drug resistance play in ear infections? Antibiotics have become the accepted and expected treatment for all ear infections. Some doctors think that antibiotics are harmless and might help an infection so they prescribe them frequently regardless of the problem. Some physicians have been known to prescribe antibiotics without reasonable cause, sometimes even over the phone at the request of unexamined patients. This is why many children, like Cari, have been on multiple rounds of antibiotics. When one antibiotic doesn't work, another, broader spectrum, more potent, antibiotic is tried.

This is how antibiotic-resistant bacteria are cultivated. While most bacteria causing an ear infection will be killed by the antibiotic, a few will survive and give birth to many more bacteria, which also cannot be killed by that drug. Each time a more potent drug is used, a few stronger bacteria survive. It has taken us a little over fifty years to develop some very serious bacteria in this manner.

This trend continues to get worse. Originally, penicillin was reliably effective in treating pneumococcus, the most common cause of bacterial middle ear infections. In 1997, *Patient Care Magazine* reported that about 40% of pneumococcal strains in parts of the United States are resistant to penicillin. In addition, strains of other common bacteria are becoming increasingly resistant to commonly used antibiotics.[6]

I decided that, if the doctors were not willing to listen, I would take this information to the patients. Maybe that will make a difference. I want to have antibiotics available if anyone in my family or any of my patients need antibiotics to stay alive. I would like to see other physicians think the same way. This is not a new concept. The pharmaceutical companies and the people in medicine have known what was occurring for the past fifty years.

We may still be able to stop this deadly trend. There was encouraging news reported from Finland recently in the *New England Journal of Medicine*. The amount of the bacteria streptococcal A which is already resistant to erythromycin actually decreased significantly, from 16.5% in 1992 to 8.6% in 1996, with the corresponding reduction in the use of erythromycin to treat it.[10]

It appears from this study that if we stop using these antibiotics so recklessly, we may still be able to reverse this trend of antibiotic-resistant bacteria. In addition, less use of antibiotics may well give our immune systems the opportunity to grow stronger.

But if antibiotic use continues at its current rate, there will soon come a time when we may be forced to treat bacterial infections the way we did before penicillin was discovered.

It all started with the introduction of antibiotics in the 1940s, an event that ushered in the era of the ''medicalization'' of health. With the discovery of this wonder drug, the antibiotic, we forgot what our bodies could do by themselves. Doctors and patients relinquished control of their health to medicine and the use of drugs.

The goal for health care should be to support the body's immune system so that it can develop the strength and the antibodies it needs to fight off infections on its own. There are many tools and techniques a parent can use to help a child's immune system fight off an ear or respiratory infection. These will be discussed and illustrated in later chapters.

When we don't give our bodies a chance to ''learn'' how to fight off different strains of bacteria, we become dependent on antibiotics to do the job for us. Meanwhile, the many different strains of bacteria in our environment are ''learning'' how to fight off our antibiotics. The bacteria are getting stronger while our immune systems are not. When there are no antibiotics left that can help fight off these virulent strains of bacteria, it will be up to our own immune systems to do the job for us.

Chapter 3

Understanding the Immune System

Different Types of Immunity

When we talk about immunity, we are referring to all the different mechanisms that the body has to protect us from things in the environment which are foreign to us. These foreign agents can be bacteria or viruses, or they can be foods, chemicals, weeds, dust, mold, or even drugs.

There are two different forms of immunity. One is "innate," meaning that we were born with these protectors. The other is "acquired," meaning that it is a process that occurs after we have been exposed to these foreign items in the environment.

How the Immune System Works

The immune system is actually a network of cells and organs that work together to defend the body. The human body provides an ideal environment for many organisms, and it is the immune system's job to keep these organisms out and, if they do invade, to find and destroy them.

The immune system is amazingly complex. It can recognize millions of different enemies and produce specific antibodies made up of chemicals and cells designed to kill each one of them.

The immune system is made up of an elaborate communications network containing millions of cells which pass information back and forth. When immune cells receive an alarm of an invasion, they begin to produce powerful chemicals, called antibodies. Once these antibodies are produced and the invader is successfully defeated, the antibody remains as part of the body's arsenal, preventing any future illnesses caused by that same type of bacteria or virus.

One of the most significant parts of our innate immunity arsenal is our skin. Our skin protects us from foreign agents invading our body. Whenever we have a cut, scrape, or deep wound, we run the risk of bacteria and viruses invading our body and making us sick. But even if that occurs, we have many other innate protectors standing guard. Our mucous membranes, the mucous that is released from them, and the cough reflex also stand ready to protect us. Fever is part of the body's innate defense system. We also have the ability to release many different chemicals which can attack, kill, or subdue an invading microorganism. Our lymph system is another innate part of our immune system. Lymph nodes lie in clusters throughout our bodies. The lymph system helps trap foreign bodies and develops the antibodies which can attack the foreign substances on their second visit into the body. All of these wonderful things came with the package. We were born with them.

In addition to our innate protectors, we have acquired ones. Acquired immunity does not start until we are exposed to something that our body reads as foreign. If the body thinks something is foreign, it will begin a process in which certain cells are activated, forming proteins. These proteins, called antibodies, fight off the infection. After a successful battle against the invader, the antibodies are ready if that same foreign body ever invades again. Our use of vaccinations is based on this idea. Vaccinations are mild forms of a disease, enough to cause us to form antibodies, but not potent enough to make us very sick. When a vaccinated individual is later exposed to the strong form of bacteria or virus which causes the disease, a defense system is already in place.

This is "acquired" immunity, and it is actually a "learned" system. Through exposures to bacteria, viruses, and other immunological factors, our immune system learns how to react. If it reacts successfully the first time the body is exposed to one of these factors, it will continue to react successfully to subsequent exposures. For example, if you are exposed to the chicken pox virus and actually get chicken pox, the next time you are exposed to the chicken pox virus, you will not get it again. Your body has learned how to react. Your immune system will now kill off the chicken pox virus. There are many different viruses and bacteria which your body is exposed to each day, and each day your immune system fights them.

Our immune system is not a perfect system, however. Sometimes it needs help, but many of the things we do in an effort to stop infections actually interfere with the immune system's ability to work properly.

What do doctors recommend when you have an upper respiratory infection and complain of fever, runny nose, and cough? You might be prescribed acetaminophen to reduce your fever, a decongestant to stop the runny nose, a cough suppressant to stop the cough, and an antibiotic to kill the bacteria. Even without a doctor, you might go to the drugstore and purchase all of those items except the antibiotic. If you take them, think about what you have just done. You have stopped practically every one of your innate immune system protectors from working. The fever might have burned out the bacteria, the mucous may have washed it out, and the cough might have removed it from your respiratory tract. If you had not used the antibiotic, your body may then have had the opportunity to wage its own battle and develop those proteins which would be on guard in the case of any future invasions. If an antibiotic is prescribed at the onset of an illness, the antibiotic will take over the immune system's job, killing the bacteria. The immune system does not get the opportunity to learn how to do the job itself. This is like a child who never learns to speak because the parents provide all the child's needs without her speaking. If she is given everything she wants or needs just because she points to something, she will have no need to develop speech. She will only learn to speak when speech is required for her to function.

The immune system will only develop when it is needed to, when there is a challenge to the immune system itself. If the antibiotic takes over the job, the immune system will never learn what to do. By doing all of the typical things we have been taught to do for infections, we may actually stop our body's defense system from working altogether. I believe this is why the sooner antibiotics are given to children who have ear infections, the longer the infections last and the more recurrences there are. I call this "The Antibiotic/Ear and Respiratory Infection Cycle" (*see* Figure 2).

How Antibiotics Can Interfere with the Immune System

It may seem strange that antibiotics, which are designed to aid the body's immune system, could actually make the problem worse, but when you take an antibiotic at the first sign of illness, the antibiotic may not give your immune system the opportunity to set up its defenses. The next time the bug comes along, your immune system is still unarmed and unprepared to battle this enemy.

It is time to take another look at how we treat illness in the United States. The very symptoms that we call illness may just be our immune system using all it has available

Figure 2

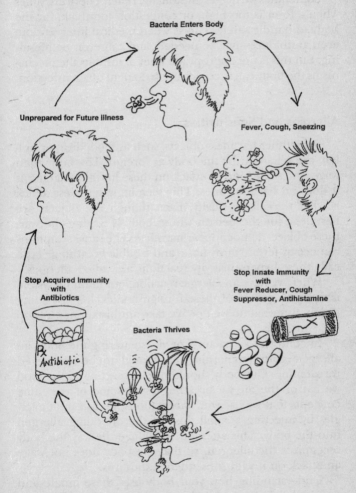

Bacteria Enters Body

Unprepared for Future Illness

Fever, Cough, Sneezing

Stop Acquired Immunity
with
Antibiotics

Rx
Antibiotic

Stop Innate Immunity
with
Fever Reducer, Cough
Suppressor, Antihistamine

Bacteria Thrives

to keep us well. A runny nose is not an illness. A runny nose is actually the way our body treats an illness or keeps us from becoming ill. It is the same with a fever or a cough.

Sometimes we need symptomatic relief. There are times when a fever is too high, or congestion too thick, for the body to handle safely. This is when medical intervention, even antibiotics, may be needed, and can even be lifesaving. But this is not appropriate when it inhibits the mechanisms the body can successfully use to fight off an infection.

Allergies and Sensitivities

Sometimes harmless objects, such as food, dust, or pollen, are regarded by the body as foreign. The body then wages the same kind of attack on these harmless agents as it does on harmful ones. This seemingly senseless attack is what we call sensitivity. Even though the objects are harmless, for the person whose body is waging the war, these objects do not appear harmless. The same symptoms can occur: fever, runny nose, and trouble breathing. Typically these hypersensitivity reactions are called allergies.

When we have an allergic reaction, our immune system is trying to get rid of these foreign bodies. It's just doing its job. But what do we do? We take antihistamines to stop the symptoms.

In contrast to a bacteria or virus entering the body, an allergen is often something that should not be considered threatening. Our body should not be reacting to the food we eat or the air we breathe. Using some of the same concepts that we use with vaccinations, we can treat allergies by injecting a small dose of the offending allergen into the body. This attempts to change the way the body recognizes the allergen, so that the body does not wage an attack on it with subsequent exposures.

Understanding how your body uses these innate and acquired defenses can help unravel the mysterious cycle of ear infections. When a foreign material, such as a bacteria or virus, is introduced into the body, the first protective response, the innate immunity, is triggered and becomes active. The first signs of this innate immunity becoming active are often fever and mucous. When parents or doctors prescribe medications to stop the fever and the mucous, the innate immunity functions are shut down. At this point, the body's second method of defense, its system of acquired immunity, will kick in to fight off the bacteria or virus. When an antibiotic is prescribed at this juncture, the acquired immunity may also be shut down, leaving the body defenseless. It is a vicious cycle.

Chapter 4

Understanding the Ear

Dissecting the Ear

Since an ear infection often has bacteria associated with it, one would think that using an antibiotic would be treating the underlying cause, but I don't think that is the case. I do not think the ear infection was caused by bacteria wandering around the body and deciding to take up residence in the ear. There has to be a reason why the bacteria are able to grow in the ear in the first place. Understanding the ear can help us find and treat the real cause of ear infections.

The common denominator in children's ear infections is the ear itself. More specifically, the structure of the ear.

The ear is a complex organ with three parts: the inner ear, the middle ear, and the outer ear. The outer ear includes the part outside the head and the ear canal. The eardrum, or tympanic membrane, is a small circle of tissue, about the size of a fingertip, at the end of the ear canal. The middle ear is the space behind the eardrum, usually filled with air. A small tube, called the eustachian tube, connects the middle ear to the back of the nose, and three tiny bones (malleus, incus, and stapes) connect the

Figure 3

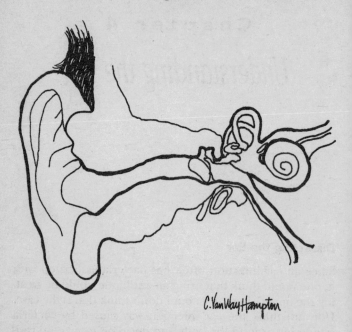

C. Van Way Hampton

eardrum, through the middle ear, to the inner ear. The inner ear, further inside the head, is important for both hearing and balance. *(See* Figure 3.)

Children Are More Susceptible to Ear Infections

A child's anatomy is different from an adult's. The eustachian tube, connecting the nose and throat to the ear, is more horizontal in a child. In an adult it is more vertical *(see* Figure 4). It is easier for fluids to drain from the adult ear through the eustachian tube because of this. This is why I can safely say that a child will almost always outgrow ear infections. Ear infections are very rare in

Figure 4

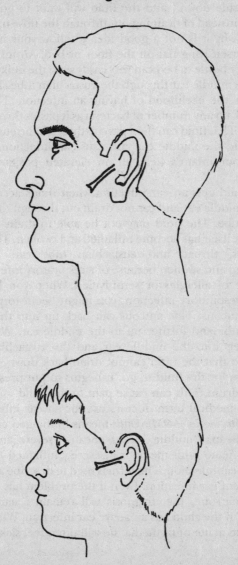

adults. If a child lies on her back, the eustachian tube will be "upside down" and the fluid will want to go toward the ear instead of draining out through the nose or throat. This is why it is not a good idea to allow your infant to feed herself lying flat on the floor or bed. An infant that takes her bottle to bed can very easily send the milk upward into the middle ear through the eustachian tube. This can increase the likelihood of having an infection. The fluid can pick up any number of bacteria as it passes through the mouth. That fluid can then pass up through the eustachian tube into the middle ear and cause an infection. Always keep your infant's head in an elevated position while feeding.

A child gets an ear infection when fluids accumulate in the middle ear and cannot drain out through the eustachian tube. The fluid may not be able to drain because the tube itself has become inflamed and swollen. The nasal passages, throat, and eustachian tube can become inflamed and swollen because of a respiratory infection or because of allergies or sensitivities. When you have an upper respiratory infection, you might begin to produce thick mucous. This mucous can back up into the eustachian tube and further up to the middle ear. When the fluid gets into the middle ear and the eustachian tube swells so that the fluid cannot drain back down, there is nowhere for the fluid to go. It begins to put pressure on the eardrum. This can cause pain to the child.

The medical term doctors use for an ear infection is *acute otitis media (AOM)*. *Otitis* means "inflamed ear" and *media* means "middle." *Acute* means "severe and short term." Acute otitis media is a severely inflamed (or red) middle ear infection. The term is used to describe an active or current ear infection. Even if the problem has become a chronic one, the diagnosis will remain "acute otitis media" if the child has an active ear infection. When your child has acute otitis media, he will often feel sick, have a fever, and may have ear pain. Other symptoms of AOM are irritability, sleep interruptions, and hearing loss.

Sometimes a child will not actually have an infection, but will have fluid in the middle ear. The fluid can cause painful bulging of the eardrum. Fluid in the ear can lead to an infection. When there is no infection, just fluid, the doctor refers to this as *otitis media with effusion (OME)*. The term *effusion* means "fluid." Other terms doctors might use include *glue* ear or *serous otitis media*.

Otitis media with effusion may actually be *acute,* in the sense that there is sudden onset, and it is active and current. It may be associated with ear pain as well. Acute otitis media or otitis media with effusion may occur in one or both ears at the same time. Acute otitis media may be considered "persistent" if the signs and symptoms do not resolve, even with treatment, after ten to fourteen days, or if the signs and symptoms recur within a short time after a successful treatment. Some use the term *recurrent* acute otitis media if a child has at least three infections within a six-month period, or five within a year.[15] Cari had both recurrent and persistent ear infections. She had been taking antibiotics for most of her life because her ear infections would not stop.

A Breeding Ground

This warm fluid in the middle ear is a wonderful place for bacteria and viruses to grow. As they do, the body produces more fluid in an attempt to wash out the bacteria and viruses. This causes further buildup in the middle ear, and more pain, because the pain is from the fluid buildup, not from the bacteria or virus. Now a vicious cycle can occur. The more fluid, the more bacteria, the more bacteria, the more fluid. Having fluid in the ear can encourage the growth of the bacteria and viruses, and having the bacteria can cause the increase of the fluid. Anything that causes the eustachian tube to become inflamed and swollen can also lead to ear infections. It can be allergies, sensitivities, tobacco smoke, colds, or even fragrances. *(See* Chapter 7.)

Sometimes the eardrum will burst, allowing the fluid to flow out. There is usually pain or discomfort when this occurs. But as soon as the membrane has burst, the pain usually resolves. Before we had antibiotics to treat ear infections, this bursting of the tympanic membrane was the usual way for an infection or effusion to resolve itself. The membrane would then heal by itself.

What Is the Underlying Cause?

The sooner you take an antibiotic for an ear infection, the longer the infection will last and the more recurrences you will have. If this is the case, why are we using antibiotics to such an extent and with such frequency? The pharmaceutical companies like it this way. When doctors prescribe drugs, drug companies profit. That doesn't mean it is the best thing for the patient. Keep in mind that prescribing drugs is what doctors do best. This is what they have been trained to do. Most have not been trained to use the treatments I am going to discuss in the next part of this book. They are trained to use a prescription pad to cover up the symptoms of a problem.

The body has an amazing capacity to heal itself if we just give it a little time to do so. But we are always in such a hurry. We want the problem to be gone now! Not next week or even tomorrow, but now! So we go to the doctor and ask for a "miracle" cure. But these cures, these prescriptions, don't cure the problem; they just cover up the symptoms.

But the antibiotic kills the bacteria, you're probably thinking. Doesn't that cure the problem? Is the bacteria really the underlying cause of the ear infection?

Let's take another look. Perhaps the real underlying

cause is the fluid buildup. If there is no fluid, the bacteria has nowhere to grow. If the eustachian tube is draining correctly on its own, the bacteria will just wash away. Bacteria and viruses need some stationary fluid to grow in. When the eustachian tube does not drain properly, a perfect medium develops for bacteria and viruses to grow. Once that occurs, an infection begins. An infection can cause more inflammation and swelling, and then the vicious cycle is in place. You can easily see why it is not enough just to treat the bacteria with an antibiotic. And it may not be a bacteria at all, but a virus, which will not be susceptible to an antibiotic. Even if it is a bacteria, killing it will only resolve the problem temporarily. If we are just killing the bacteria with the antibiotic, and not doing anything about draining the fluid, the bacteria will return as soon as the antibiotic is gone.

To fix the problem for the long term, we must fix the underlying cause of the problem—the swollen eustachian tube that keeps the fluid in the middle ear. If we could do something to drain the fluid, perhaps then the ear infections would go away for good.

Tubes in the Ears

Tympanostomy, or putting tubes in the ears, has become a very popular surgical procedure in the last twenty-five years. In fact, it is the most common surgery for children in the United States. In 1988, approximately 670,000 children underwent surgeries to insert tympanostomy tubes in the United States. Thirty percent of these replaced tubes had fallen out on their own.[16]

The purpose of this surgical procedure is to give the tympanic membrane a way to get rid of the fluids that have built up. The fluid simply drains out the tube. This technique appeals to common sense. If we cannot get the fluid to drain naturally down through the eustachian tube, then why not put a hole in the ear (myringotomy) and let the fluid drain out that way? This concept made sense to me before I went to medical school. It made sense to me when doctors recommended it for my eighteen-month-old son. But the concept of surgically putting a hole in a child's ear no longer makes sense to me.

There are facts every parent should consider seriously before agreeing to this operation for their child. The process of putting a hole in someone's eardrum, while it may help with one problem, could lead to an entirely new set of problems. Myringotomy with the insertion of tubes is a major surgery, which requires an anesthetic. In addition, it doesn't always work. I have seen many children who have tubes in their ears continue to have infections.

One study indicated that using tubes presented no better solution to chronic ear infections than using chronic antibiotics or even doing nothing at all![5] Also, scarring of the eardrum can occur, particularly if more than one set of tubes is needed. When scarring occurs, hearing and learning problems are more likely. Since 1985, there has been evidence that myringotomy with the insertion of tubes may lead to permanent structural damage of the eardrum, causing tissue death and hearing loss.[8]

A study in England found 87% of all children, ages two to four, who had tubes inserted for middle ear infections had structural damage of the eardrum when followed up at age eight.[17]

Another study indicated that 25% of all tube insertions may be inappropriate and that for only 30% of all cases was the benefit worth the risk.[11]

Why would we want to put a child under that risk when, if left alone, 90% of all ear infections will heal on their own? While doing nothing for an ear infection has been shown to be 90% effective, many parents find it difficult to sit back and wait. We have been trained to be active, not passive, when it comes to our children's health. Based on my own experience as a parent, I could not agree more. But if we need to be active, let's at least try techniques that don't cause more harm than good. These are the kinds of techniques I use and teach the parents of my patients.

Acute otitis media is one of the most common illnesses in childhood. Acute otitis media may manifest itself as symptomatic or as asymptomatic. The child may have no apparent symptoms like pain or fever; or she may have pain, fever, and a bright red ear with fluid in it. If asymptomatic, the ear infection may only be noticed if the child is being evaluated for some other condition.

Acute otitis media and otitis media with effusion are most common in younger children. Currently no laboratory tests are regularly done to determine if someone actually has an ear infection. Myringotomy—putting a hole in the tympanic membrane—draining the fluid, and evaluating it under a microscope are the only way to know if bacteria are actually growing, and this is rarely done. It is not acceptable practice to make a hole in the tympanic membrane just to see what kind of bacteria may be growing there. A study was conducted in 1966 to rate the value of myringotomy, and researchers concluded the procedure was an unnecessary risk. Since the cause of ear infections—mainly bacteria—can be predicted fairly well, the need for myringotomy to establish an accurate diagnosis is not warranted and does not outweigh the discomfort caused by the procedure. It does not outweigh the expense or the possible danger from giving a child general anesthesia.[18]

I agree. I do not think the information gained from myringotomy is worth the risk. In addition to the effects from anesthesia and physical pain, puncturing the eardrum can cause scarring and lead to hearing loss.

Tools of the Trade

Many parents have related to me that they would like to use an otoscope *(see* Figure 5) to look in their children's ears at home. The otoscope lights up the outer ear canal and magnifies the appearance inside the canal. Many have

Figure 5

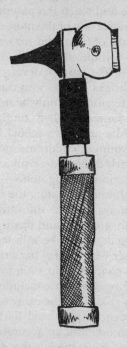

been told by their pediatricians that a parent could not possibly look at the middle ear through an otoscope and understand what they are seeing. They feel that only a trained doctor can do this. However, the parents I meet in my office could very well do this. After being told by her child's pediatrician that she would not be able to master this skill, one mother purchased her own otoscope and began observing her child's ears. She did not tell the pediatrician that she was using this tool and the pediatrician continued to be amazed at how effective she was at bringing her children in to see him at the very onset of their ear infections. The ear is a very interesting organ, but not so complex that the layperson cannot understand how it works and how fluid builds up and infections occur. There was a time when thermometers and blood pressure cuffs were considered tools of the physician only. I believe parents are quite capable of learning and understanding more specifically how to care for their children's health care.

To diagnose an ear infection, the doctor usually looks into the outer ear canal with his otoscope. The tool does not allow the doctor to look beyond the tympanic membrane, however. In addition, the physician cannot get a sample of the fluid behind the tympanic membrane with an otoscope.

Your doctor may use another test, called pneumatic otoscopy, to determine if there is fluid in the middle ear. Pneumatic otoscopy combines the visual exam of the otoscope with a test of membrane mobility. The doctor will blow air against the tympanic membrane. If the tympanic membrane does not move, or doesn't move much, there is probably fluid behind it.

Sometimes a physician can simply look into the ear canal and see a bulging eardrum. This, too, can indicate that there is fluid there. But the accuracy of the otoscope and the pneumatic otoscopy is somewhat subjective.

Even the determination of redness is somewhat subjective. As mentioned earlier, if the outside of a child's ear is red, then the inside, including the eardrum, will probably be red also. It does not mean the child has an ear infection; it just means the skin is red. If a child has been crying or has a fever, often the outside and inside of the ear will be red. If that is the case, one cannot actually diagnose an ear infection accurately.

Another instrument used to diagnose problems in the middle ear is a tympanogram. The tympanogram can determine if fluid is behind the tympanic membrane. This instrument is computerized and appears to be very accurate in determining if fluid is behind the eardrum. A tympanogram is performed by placing a probe in the ear and taking a reading off a machine. It is not invasive or painful for the child.

Since myringotomy (puncturing the eardrum) is not done, we don't really know which bacteria are responsible for the symptoms. However, it has been shown that certain antibiotics are effective against most of the likely bacteria. Amoxicillin is considered to be the first-line drug for the treatment of ear infections. It is also very cost-effective.

The timing for antibiotic treatment has been determined somewhat empirically. The number of days of treatment is also somewhat empirical. In the United States a child is usually treated for ten to fourteen days. Other countries use shorter trials. And as I've mentioned, there are studies that indicate that antibiotics may not be necessary at all.

Prevention of ear and respiratory infections would be the best route, eliminating the pain, discomfort, surgery, possible hearing loss, and cost.

What Are the First Signs of Ear Infection?

An ear infection may manifest itself with or without any symptoms at all. The child may have no apparent symptoms, or she may have pain, fever, and a bright red ear with fluid in it. Fluid may drain from the ear.

One of the first signs of a middle ear problem may be a change in your child's behavior or sleeping habits. A child may pull or tug repeatedly at the ear, or frequently poke her finger into the ear.

Symptoms of earaches commonly include:

- Ear pain
- Fever
- Drainage from the ear
- Sleeplessness
- Irritability

- Change in eating habits
- Change in hearing
- Refusal to nurse on one side
- Nasal obstruction or discharge

Another potential problem from fluid in the ear is hearing loss. Many studies have noted hearing problems caused by fluid in the ear, and the effect this loss of hearing may have on language development.

One study evaluated the effectiveness of treating ear infections with four different approaches:

1. Antibiotics
2. Myringotomy
3. Both antibiotics and myringotomy
4. Neither antibiotics nor myringotomy

This study followed 171 children and 239 infected ears that were treated with one of these four approaches, and no significant differences in outcome were determined. There were no complications associated with any of the treatments.[5]

First, Do No Harm

Most physicians are trained in what I call the drug model of practicing medicine. When drugs won't work, they often resort to surgery. This current approach should not be the only treatment available, especially to parents who are willing to work to uncover the source of illness.

Why would we want to put a child under risk from surgery or the negative effects of antibiotics when, if left alone, 90% of all ear infections will heal on their own?

Chapter 5

The Federal Guidelines

A New Set of Rules

Ear infections are so widespread that the United States government has taken a position on their treatment and causes. In 1992, a nonfederal panel of experts was formed to examine the diagnosis and treatment of otitis media with effusion or fluid in the ears. This committee was sponsored by the Agency for Health Care Policy and Research, a division of the U.S. Department of Health and Human Services. A host of agencies were involved in the panel selection, including the American Academy of Pediatrics, the American Academy of Family Physicians, and the American Academy of Otolaryngology Head and Neck Surgery. The panel's mission was to set forth guidelines for doctors, nurses, and other health care providers in diagnosing and treating ear infections in children.

Because of my experience in treating children with ear infections, I was asked to serve as a peer reviewer for this committee. I was given an opportunity to look at the findings of the panel and give my comments before the information was published.

The committee's findings were made public in 1994,

and were published in Quick Reference Guide for Clinicians, "Managing Otitis Media with Effusion in Young Children."[19] The committee findings were also published in a parent guide called "Middle Ear Fluid in Young Children." You may have received this pamphlet when visiting your doctor.

The panel's guidelines are very important because third-party insurance reimbursement is based on these standards for diagnosis and treatment. Guidelines are a good idea only if the conclusions are drawn from extensive, unbiased research. I plan to show you how the panel disregarded many proven treatments and fell into the recurring trap of limiting medical practice to the current model: drugs and surgery.

First, I'll discuss what the panel discovered. Then, I'll tell you what I and some other physicians think about the final recommendations of the panel.

Why Ear Infections Are a Serious Problem

The panel states that doctors in the United States diagnose middle ear infections more than any other disease in children younger than fifteen years. Almost all children have one or more episodes of ear infection requiring a visit to the doctor before the age of six.

Hearing loss at an early age is widely accepted as a risk factor for impaired speech and language development. In general, the earlier the hearing problem begins, the worse its effects on speech and language development. The panel noted that middle ear infections are often associated with a mild to moderate hearing loss, but found no consistent, reliable evidence that otitis media with effusion has long-term effects on language or learning.[19]

Diagnosing Ear Infections

To diagnose ear infections with fluid, the committee recommends four procedures:

1. Suspect otitis media with effusion in young children. Since most children have at least one episode of otitis media with effusion before entering school, the panel urges doctors to suspect this disease when a child shows symptoms of discomfort or behavior changes. (I wonder how many children have their ears examined before receiving a diagnosis of attention deficit hyperactivity disorder.)
2. Use pneumatic otoscopy to assess middle ear status. This instrument combines a visual examination of the tympanic membrane with a test of membrane mobility.
3. Tympanometry may be performed to confirm middle ear fluid. This test measures how well the eardrum moves as a way of determining middle ear fluid. An eardrum with fluid behind it will not move as well.
4. A child who has had fluid in both ears for a total of three months should undergo a hearing evaluation. Because surgery is not the recommended treatment in middle ear infections unless it is causing hearing loss, the panel recommends a hearing exam.[19]

Environmental Risk Factors

The panel pointed to scientific evidence linking certain environmental factors with an increased risk of getting middle ear infections:

- Bottle-feeding rather than breastfeeding infants
- Passive smoking
- Attending group child-care facilities

However, since the target child selected for this study was beyond nursing age, the panel did not delve into breastfeeding versus bottle-feeding.

Children who are exposed to smokers have a higher risk of getting middle ear infections.

Children who stay in group child-care facilities have a slightly higher risk of getting middle ear infections than children who stay at home.[19]

The Panel's Recommended Treatment Options

The panel admits that more than half of the cases of middle ear infections with fluid will heal without treatment within three months. Even after three months, the rate of healing continues at the same level, so only a very small percentage of children have fluid in the ears that last for a year or longer. The panel also notes most cases of ear infections do not last beyond early childhood.

With these facts in mind, the panel recommends the following treatments:

1. *Observation or antibiotic therapy.* The panel notes again that most cases of ear infections resolve spontaneously. The panel also refers to studies showing a 14% increase in the resolution rate of ear fluid when antibiotics were prescribed. The panel does make mention of the adverse effects of antibiotics, the most common being stomach and skin disorders. The guidelines did not mention that a study published in the *Journal of the American Medical Association* in 1991 indicates that treating fluid in the ear with antibiotics is inappropriate. The panel recommended observation or antibiotics for treatment when children have had middle ear fluid for less than four to six months and no discernible hearing loss.

2. *Surgery to insert tubes.* Although the panel could find no studies identifying long-term negative effects of fluid in the ears, they were concerned that long-term consequences could occur. This concern led them to recommend surgery. Surgery is targeted by the panel as a treatment for

ear fluid when a child has had fluid in the ear and a hearing loss for a total of four to six months.

The panel does note risks for two specific complications of surgery: 51% may experience tympanosclerosis, or scarring of the tympanic membrane, and 13% may experience postoperative otorrhea, or ear pain. This points to a 64% chance of postsurgery complications. It did not point out that some studies indicate that children receiving tubes may do no better than those who don't.

The panel also listed numerous treatments that they do not recommend for fluid in the ear, including steroids, antihistamines, decongestants, adenoidectomy (surgery to remove the adenoids), tonsillectomy (surgery to remove the tonsils), allergy treatment, and "alternative therapies."[19]

What the Federal Guidelines Miss

The panel's position on allergies deserves a review. The guidelines state, "The association between allergy and otitis media with effusion was not clear from available evidence. Thus, although close anatomic relationships between the nasopharynx, eustachian tube, and middle ear have led many experts to suggest a role for allergy management in treating otitis media with effusion, no recommendation was made for or against such treatment."[19]

In my practice alone, I have encountered numerous cases where allergies played a significant role in ear infections. There are many other scientific studies available which link allergies to middle ear infections. I can't imagine why the panel disregarded the evidence.

Alternative Treatments Were Completely Disregarded

The panel lumped all alternative therapies in one category, and wrote off these treatment methods as ineffective.

"Evidence regarding other therapies for the treatment of otitis media with effusion was sought, but no reports of chiropractic, holistic, naturopathic, traditional/indigenous, homeopathic, or other treatments contained information obtained in randomized controlled studies. Therefore, no recommendation was made regarding such therapies for the treatment of otitis media with effusion in children."[19]

In other words, because double-blind studies could not be performed on these treatments, the panel could not give existing research any validity. If you consider some of the treatments targeted, you'll see why this approach has faults. There is no way to conduct a double-blind study to measure the effectiveness of treatments in which the patient, or the patient's parent, is a knowing participant in the process.

As I explained earlier, double-blind studies are biased toward drug therapies, and in many treatments, a double-blind study is out of the question. In rating the effectiveness of chiropractic care, a patient would most certainly know whether he or she had received a treatment, and the doctor would know whether or not she had administered a treatment.

Before pharmaceutical companies started studies to measure drug effectiveness, the double-blind study was not considered the benchmark against which all other studies are measured. Now, for many, the double-blind study is the only method of ensuring accurate results. This is a great misfortune.

Many other physicians have greeted the clinical guidelines for otitis media with effusion in young children with the same skepticism as I have.

In a commentary published in the *American Academy of Pediatrics Newsletter*, Quentin Van Meter, M.D., F.A.A.P., takes a stand against the federal recommendations for middle ear fluid. He points out that there are certain interventions this particular panel did not approve of but which they had no research to refute. He continues, "The heft of each recommendation, then, rested on the personal opinion of the panel, and not on peer reviewed, bona fide clinical research."[20]

Dr. Van Meter also questions the selection of panel members, which included two physicians in private practice (one pediatrician and one family practitioner), four academic otolaryngologists (doctors in a university setting, and not practicing regularly), two academic family practitioners, and one academic pediatrician. The rest of the panel consisted of allied health personnel. The fact that there were very few physicians from private practice could have influenced the panel's findings. Dr. Van Meter harshly states, "To allow the 'strong opinion of the panel,' backed by only limited scientific evidence, to dictate the way I practice medicine is *bad medicine.*"

My personal reactions to the panel's guidelines are mixed. When I first read the original guidelines which were sent to me for review, I was extremely disappointed. The recommendations were no different from what doctors had been doing for years—antibiotics and then tubes if the antibiotics did not work. The revised guidelines, which I did not review prior to their publication, gave a few more options. First, antibiotics became an option rather than a "must." The published guidelines did leave room for individual doctor-patient decision-making. However, I did not feel that the panel did an adequate job of researching the literature for treatment options. I had sent them a great deal of information from the osteopathic literature on treating ear infections and fluid. That information did not become part of the guidelines. There appeared to be a double standard as to what went into the guidelines and what was left out. If the panel decided to put a recommendation into the guidelines, it did not matter if there was documentation to support it. If they decided to leave something out, "lack of documentation" was cited as the reason. I would have liked to have seen some consistency in those decisions.

I agree with Dr. Van Meter: If there are going to be guidelines, they need to be consistent. If there is not enough information to make an appropriate decision, then no decision should be made. They stated that there was insufficient data to say that allergies could affect fluid in the ear, so allergy treatment was not considered part of the protocol. But then the panel went on to say that there was also insufficient data to state that chronic fluid affected hearing or development later in life, but still recommended a child have tubes placed in the ear if the child had hearing loss in both ears for three months. I happen to think that fluid in the ear can have an adverse effect on a child's hearing and development later in life. That is another one of those "commonsense" things, but it is the inconsistency of the decisions that concerns me.

In summary, I do not think that there was enough information available for the panel to make much of any determination on the diagnosis and treatment for fluid in the ears. There is presently too much conflicting data in the medical literature. Unfortunately, the guidelines reflect only the biases of the panel. If guidelines are needed, we should do our homework first. Maybe the government should sponsor research for all of these treatment methods. Let's spend the money to find out which ones really work. Only then should we even think about setting up guidelines.

PART II

How I Treat Ear and Respiratory Infections without Antibiotics or Tubes

The Block System for Treating Ear and Respiratory Infections is very simple to learn. Any parent can do it. In fact, after I teach it to parents, they often tell me that they then use it on everyone in the family, not just the child who was originally brought in to see me. Please, learn the treatment and use it on everyone. There is no age limit. When I produced a videotape of the treatment protocol, one of the men who was producing the video said he began using the treatment on his girlfriend and "It really worked!" The treatment is multidisciplined, and one of the most important components is gentle osteopathic manipulation.

Chapter 6

Osteopathic Medicine

A New Medicine

In the late 1800s, Andrew Taylor Still founded a medical model and philosophy. This model was, for the most part, based on Hippocrates' concept that the body had an inherent ability to heal itself. Dr. Still also studied anatomy intensely and found that, in order to heal, it was important that the paths of blood vessels and nerves be unimpeded. Otherwise, he believed, healing could not occur and disease would follow. Dr. Still also believed we had all the drugs we needed in our own bodies already. He said that "Man should study and use the drugs compounded in his own body."

He called his model osteopathy. Though the "specific etiology" model (the drug model) was already in place when Dr. Still developed this new concept, osteopathic medicine was able to establish itself even in this opposing environment.

The medicines of the day were generally purges and leeches. Dr. Still's methods were less traumatic and destructive to the body, and more importantly, they worked. By 1918 when the dreadful flu epidemic swept this country, thousands of people were dying from the flu or from pneumonia. History has recorded that patients with influenza and pneumonia who were treated by osteopathic physicians with osteopathic manipulation (OMT) survived in greater numbers than those who were treated by M.D.s. Osteopathy gained notoriety and popularity because of its effectiveness. But osteopathy's glory was not to last. Enter the miracle drugs, antibiotics.

The introduction of antibiotics into the medical arena confirmed the "specific etiology" model as the "true" medical model, and drugs as the "true" defense. This ushered in a new era of pharmaceuticals in medicine and solidly established the drug model, which still dominates today.

Even though osteopathy would remain as a medical philosophy, and the profession continued to grow, it would never again reach the pinnacle of glory it had attained during those few short years. Pharmaceutical companies took this advantage and ran with it, taking over medicine and never looking back. These companies have grown into a massive industry, woven into our economic and medical systems. It is no wonder the primary treatment for ear infections is antibiotics. There is no question that drugs bring enormous benefits to the quality of our lives, but there is also a darker side to this drug model—serious side effects as well as abuse and overuse. If the predictions about drug resistance come true, we will be right back where we were in 1918, without the use of antibiotics. If we are ever in that position again, I certainly want my doctor to know how to use OMT.

What is OMT?

Osteopathic Manipulation Treatment (OMT) is something that is often misunderstood by the public. I know I certainly misunderstood it before I took my daughter Michelle to an osteopathic physician many years ago. I had always been biased against osteopathic physicians. Though they are fully licensed to practice medicine, I thought they were simply not as good as "real" doctors, M.D.s. If you read my first book, *No More Ritalin,* you already know about my former bias. Because of this bias, I was skeptical about taking my daughter to an osteopath when she was ill. However, I had taken her to see many M.D.s, and not only had none of them helped, but some had actually made the problem worse. So I decided to try an osteopath.

When this osteopath suggested, on our first visit, that he would like to do some osteopathic manipulation on my daugher, I said, "Over my dead body." Having run into this sort of bias before, the doctor did not press me. Instead, he began to explain what OMT was all about and how it worked. I thought OMT was all about bones, spinal alignment, and "popping and cracking" the neck. I was certainly wrong about that. There are many very gentle OMT treatments available to the osteopath who wishes to avail herself of them.

Shared Responsibility

On our initial visit I let him know that I was tired of dealing with doctors who would not listen to me, doctors who discounted what I knew about my own child. I had no time or energy to talk to or work with a doctor who would not let me help make medical decisions about my child. I was angry about the experiences I had had with doctors before meeting this osteopath. I was mad about the doctors who had misused medications and caused my child to be sick for three years, then claimed that her problems were all in her head. I was only interested in working with a doctor who saw me as a partner. If he could not do that, then I had nothing else to say to him. This wonderful doctor just nodded and said that was fine with him. His entire approach was based on the patient being part of the equation. He believed that, as a physician, his job was to educate the patient. He could not do much to get the patient well if the patient did not wish to do so. He did not have a problem with my participating in the process; in fact, he expected it.

At the second visit, Michelle was using crutches. She had such severe allergic reactions to mosquito bites that her legs would swell and she could not walk around without crutches. This swelling and discomfort would continue for days. Michelle had just been stung and the swelling had just begun when we entered the doctor's office that day. He immediately said that Michelle needed some OMT to help reduce the swelling and assist the body in removing the mosquito toxin from her system. He explained how he would gently perform this treatment. I felt I could trust this man who had shown me a different approach to medicine, so I let him perform OMT on my daughter.

The treatment was indeed very gentle. Shortly after he finished, the swelling of Michelle's mosquito bites began to lessen, and within a few hours, they were gone. She no longer needed the crutches to walk. This was incredible. This OMT treatment had a dramatic effect on Michelle's legs. It normally would have taken at least a week for this same resolution of the bites. I was thrilled! Not only had we found a doctor who I felt I could trust, but it also appeared that he could perform miracles. What he had actually done was to use an old, well-established tool which is not well known or understood in our current medical model. Yet it was more effective than all the drugs doctors had given Michelle for this problem. Soon after, I became his patient myself. I let him treat an old back injury that had never completely resolved. He was able to successfully treat my back as well.

Eureka!

As our new doctor continued to work with Michelle and relieve her ongoing health problems, I continued to be impressed with the way he practiced medicine. I wondered how osteopathic medicine had escaped the public's knowledge. Not only did most people not even know the profession existed, but most of those who did had biases similar to mine. I was so taken with what I perceived as osteopathic medicine and had such a strong desire to ensure that what had happened to Michelle would never happen to anyone I loved again, that I decided to become an osteopathic physician. I went back to school and took the prerequisites for medical school, took the entrance exam, and applied to the Texas College of Osteopathic Medicine. In August 1984, at the age of thirty-nine, I walked through the door as a medical student, expecting to find many more doctors like our doctor on the other side. Boy, was I in for a surprise!

A D.O. Is Not Necessarily an Osteopath

While our doctor was practicing the very best of osteopathic medicine, I found that many doctors who had gone to osteopathic medical schools did so just to become doctors, not because they wanted to practice osteopathic medicine. I found that many on the faculty took no pride in their profession and would rather have been M.D.s. While I enjoyed learning OMT in medical school, many did not. They thought it was a waste of time, something they would never use as a doctor. These students ultimately graduated from the same medical school I did, but we were very different. They received the D.O. degree, but I felt that I had become an "osteopath."

Many patients who have been to me, or another osteopathic physician like me, have told me they want to use only osteopaths as their doctors. I tell them to be sure they pick an osteopath, not just a D.O. There are many fine M.D.s who are actually very osteopathic in their thinking and approach. We should not judge someone just by the letters after their name, as I once did.

Gentle OMT

I was convinced in one short office visit that OMT could work wonders. Osteopathic physicians have many different modalities of OMT treatments available to them. Some use only the popping and cracking. That was all they learned when they were in school, or it was all they wanted to learn. Some doctors like the popping and cracking because the treatment may seem more obvious to the patient. You can hear the "pop." I prefer the gentler techniques myself. When using OMT on children, I find the gentle techniques work very well and do not scare the child or the parent. I remember how I used to feel about OMT and find that many of the parents I work with have similar concerns. Using gentle treatments usually removes those concerns. If the treatment works and the child gets better without any trauma, everyone is happier.

I discovered my protocol for ear and respiratory infections some time ago. It combines OMT treatments I learned in school with other modalities that I learned in other classes. I believe that the biggest problem we have concerning ear and respiratory infections is all of the excess fluid in the head that gives the bacteria and virus a place to grow. To rid the body of the bacteria or virus, we must rid it of the fluid. We must be able to have our immune system working at its best. This is the basis of my OMT treatment. It is a treatment which helps to drain the fluids from the head and neck and helps the immune system work better.

No More Surgery for Seth

Seth was only seven years old when his mother brought him to see me. He had been suffering with recurring sinus infections for several years, and recurring tonsillitis before that. When doctors removed his tonsils, the infections simply moved from the tonsils to the sinuses. He had already undergone sinus surgery, which had not been successful. When traditional medicine fails, it often tries to use the same tools again and again. So it was with Seth.

Having no other tools available, his doctor recommended doing another sinus surgery. Not knowing there was another option, his mother agreed, even though the first one was ineffective. His insurance company approved the second procedure. Before proceeding, though, his mother brought her son to me for another opinion. I treated Seth with The Block System for Treating Ear and Respiratory Infections and taught it to his mother. Seth was not sick again for many years and he did not need another surgery. His insurance company, which paid for an expensive sinus surgery that did not work, and was willing to pay for a second expensive sinus surgery in spite of its poor track record, refused to pay for the successful OMT treatments, which were less expensive than the surgery.

The osteopathic philosophy states that "the body has an inherent ability to heal itself." As an osteopathic physician, my goal is to help each patient find and treat the underlying cause of their symptoms. It does no good in the long run to simply treat symptoms. The problem will just continue to return.

OMT and Ear and Respiratory Infections

There are several treatment modalities used to treat ear and respiratory infections with OMT. D.O.s learn many different methods. One is the popping and cracking, otherwise known as "high velocity/low amplitude." This treatment is not used in my protocol. Others are muscle energy, cranial, trigger band, effleurage, strain/counterstrain, and lymphatic pump. Though many who treat ear infections use cranial treatments, cranial work is not something I can teach parents in a few minutes. I have also found that it is rarely necessary to use cranial for the treatment of ear and respiratory infections. My protocol uses the last three mentioned: strain/counterstrain, effleurage, and lymphatic pump. They will be demonstrated in the last chapter.

Strain/Counterstrain

Strain/counterstrain is a technique originated by Larry Jones, D.O. Dr. Jones had become frustrated while working with a patient. He had not been able to help this man with any of the treatments he normally used. As he moved the man around into various positions, his nurse interrupted him to take an important phone call. Dr. Jones left his patient for a few minutes in a position in which he was comfortable. The patient had noted that this particular position was about the only way he found relief from his pain. When Dr. Jones returned from the phone call, he moved the patient out of that position, and found the man was no longer in pain. Dr. Jones then spent many years determining which types of positions could relieve which type of pain.

Simply stated, he found that by shortening a muscle that was sore or pulled, it seemed to send a message to the brain that there was no more pain for which the brain needed to be concerned. In this manner, the pain ceased. This is one of my favorite treatments as it is easy and safe to perform. It is also very successful. It makes sense physiologically as well.

Sometimes we don't completely understand why a particular treatment works; we just know it does. In the osteopathic profession, we not only know that strain/counterstrain works, but we also know how it works. I am teaching you how to use this treatment to help with ear and respiratory infections, but it is a treatment that is also useful for pulled or sore muscles.

The Lymphatic Pump

The lymphatic pump is another of my favorite treatments. It is the one first used on Michelle, the one that caused the swelling from her mosquito bites to vanish. The lymphatic pump is one of the few treatments that has actually been validated in research. The first reference in the osteopathic medical literature about the lymphatic pump was in 1910. There has been information in the medical literature several times since. Consistently found was an increase in the white cells' ability to kill bacteria and increased antibodies against specific cells. The lymphatic pump can contribute to the ability of our acquired immunity. John Measel, Ph.D., published his studies on the lymphatic pump in 1982. He found that there was definitely a difference in the results with those treated with the lymphatic pump versus those who were not. His work suggests that the lymphatic pump has an effect on the B-cell component of the immune response.[21] I saw the effects on my daughter with my own eyes, and with many patients since. Osteopaths have used the lymphatic pump for at least eighty-five years because it has such a positive impact on the immune system. I wonder why it was overlooked in the federal guidelines on fluid in the ear.

In 1920, C. E. Miller, D.O., suggested that the lymphatic pump allowed for a favorable response in patients with influenza, bronchitis, pneumonia, tonsillitis, scarlet fever, and chicken pox.[22] Perhaps it was the treatment with the lymphatic pump that proved crucial in the successful OMT treatment during the influenza epidemic of 1918.

When I was an intern, a pediatrician came to me and asked me to treat a patient with pneumonia. This was an unusual request because the pediatricians at my hospital fell more into the D.O. category than the osteopathic, and rarely considered the use of OMT on their patients. I even overheard one pediatrician say that "OMT has no place in pediatrics." The pediatrician asked me to treat this baby because "we have done all we know how to do and this child is not getting any better."

The baby had been in the hospital for five days with pneumonia with no improvement. I treated the baby with the lymphatic pump and the child was released for home the very next day. The pediatrician told me that the child's x-ray was 70% better after my treatment.

I thought this would mean the other doctors in the hospital, who did not use OMT, would finally recognize its benefits. Sadly, this was not to be. This same pediatrician did ask me to treat that same baby about one year later when he returned to the hospital for the same problem. That time, the child was able to go home in two days. But I was never again asked to treat any other child with pneumonia.

I did get to treat one more child with the lymphatic pump during my internship. I was in the emergency room with a physician when we admitted a young girl into the hospital. The girl had an inflammation of the lymph gland in her neck. Upon admission, I asked the doctor for permission to treat the girl with the lymphatic pump. He denied my request. I nagged him frequently to allow me to treat the girl throughout her stay in the hospital. Each time he said "No." Finally, after several days of IV antibiotic treatment with no improvement, I found this doctor scratching his head outside the child's room. He did not understand why she was not getting better. I once again asked to be allowed to treat her with the lymphatic pump. Finally, with a huge sigh, he said "OK." Within thirty minutes the girl's neck swelling improved, and by the next morning it was gone. She was released from the hospital that day.

OMT and Scientific Proof

Osteopathic manipulation is one of those treatments which doesn't fall easily into the double-blind study criteria. Previously, all medical treatments were expected to undergo double-blind crossover placebo studies to prove their efficacy. Any treatment that could not pass this test was considered to be invalid. However, this was applied only to treatments that conventional medicine did not want to accept. Surgery is rarely validated by a double-blind study, yet surgeries are a very accepted part of mainstream medicine. The argument is that, after the surgery, you can see the outcome. This argument seems to be reserved for surgery only since there are many other treatments, including OMT, that have good outcomes.

Never mind that patients feel better and can function better after an OMT treatment. OMT has not jumped through the specific hoops that conventional medicine expects it to jump through; therefore it could not possibly be valid.

With pressure from patients who want rational use of medicine, and the HMOs which require a whole new set of hoops to jump through, the medical establishment is beginning to see that this approach does not make a lot of sense. Doctors used to make money by seeing sick people in their office. Now they make money by keeping the patient out of the office. Doctors are becoming a little more open to treatments which can help keep their patients well and out of their clinics. Now outcome studies are becoming more acceptable.

My Protocol Has Good Treatment Results

In my outcome study of sixteen patients who received my protocol for chronic ear infections, 100% got well. Most had their ear problems resolve within three weeks of beginning the treatment. These were children who had previously been treated conventionally for months, and even years.

More recently I have been able to document my success treating ear infections with OMT by using a tympanogram. I test the child with the tympanogram first, then show the parents how to do the OMT treatment. After a full treatment has been done on the child, I repeat the tympanogram. Often it takes more than one OMT treatment to see the changes on the tympanogram, but below is an example of one dramatic improvement.

Edward, an eight-month-old, has a story similar to Cari's: Chronic ear infections with chronic use of antibiotics. Doctors had recommended tubes. The parents were concerned about so much antibiotic use and really did not want to put their baby under an anesthetic for surgery to put a hole in his ear. I did a base line tympanogram on Edward during his first office visit. When we redid the tympanogram after one treatment, the tympanogram graph went from almost flat to almost normal. *(See* Figure 6.) I rechecked Edward one week later and saw him again a few weeks after that. His mother called six months later to tell me that he was still doing well and had not had another ear infection nor needed another round of antibiotics.

Effleurage Treatment

Effleurage is another very simple OMT treatment. It involves simply moving the fluids in the head, the neck, and the rest of the body to encourage proper drainage, and to help the lymph system work better. Osteopaths learn a lot about the lymph system. As mentioned in Chapter 3, the lymph system is responsible for removing the toxins from the body. If the lymph system is not working properly, our immune system is not working properly. Combining the lymphatic pump and effleurage in a single treatment allows the lymph system to improve its functioning.

Figure 6

THE BLOCK CENTER

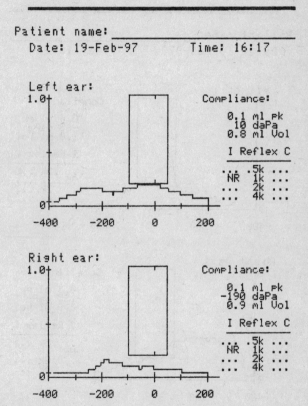

Patient name: _____

Date: 19-Feb-97   Time: 16:17

Left ear:
1.0

Compliance:

0.1 ml Pk
10 daPa
0.8 ml Vol

I Reflex C

```
···  .5k  ···
 NR  1k  ···
···  2k  ···
···  4k  ···
```

Right ear:
1.0

Compliance:

0.1 ml Pk
-190 daPa
0.9 ml Vol

I Reflex C

```
···  .5k  ···
 NR  1k  ···
···  2k  ···
···  4k  ···
```

American Electromedics Corp.
AE-206 Tympanometer Serial #261850
Calibration date: 27-Nov-94

Tester: _T. Campbell, MA_
Comments:

Figure 6 (continued)

THE BLOCK CENTER

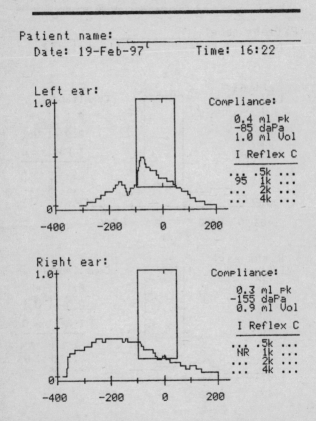

Patient name: _____
  Date: 19-Feb-97   Time: 16:22

Left ear:
1.0+

Compliance:

0.4 ml Pk
-85 daPa
1.0 ml Vol

I Reflex C

... .5k ...
95 1k ...
... 2k ...
... 4k ...

-400   -200   0   200

Right ear:
1.0+

Compliance:

0.3 ml Pk
-155 daPa
0.9 ml Vol

I Reflex C

... .5k ...
NR 1k ...
... 2k ...
... 4k ...

-400   -200   0   200

American Electromedics Corp.
AE-206 Tympanometer Serial #261850
Calibration date: 27-Nov-94

Tester: _Terri Campbell, MA._
Comments:

Remember, "the body has the ability to heal itself." We must help put everything in place so it can do so. It is not enough to depend only on OMT to accomplish this goal. It is also important to identify and eliminate irritants to our system which can cause a whole range of health problems, including ear and respiratory infections.

Chapter 7

Allergies and Sensitivities

Allergies and Ear and Respiratory Infections

Laura had chronic ear infections and had been on continuous antibiotics for nearly two years. Her parents were tired of this endless routine—another infection, another round of antibiotics. As soon as she was over one round of antibiotics, another ear infection would occur and she'd be back on antibiotics again. Her parents were concerned. They felt that antibiotic use like this could not be good for their daughter.

We identified the foods and other elements to which Laura was allergic, so that she could avoid them. I also showed them how to do The Block System for Treating Ear and Respiratory Infections, and Laura stayed well for a very long time. The next time I saw them, they were concerned that Laura had another ear infection. The day before, their babysitter had given Laura one of the foods to which she was sensitive. Laura had awakened at 3:00 A.M. crying and saying her ear hurt. Instead of calling me in the middle of the night, her parents began my OMT protocol on Laura. In a few minutes Laura was back to sleep. When she awoke the next morning, she appeared fine, but her parents brought her in to see me just to be sure. A look in the ears revealed no redness, no fluid, no problem. I spoke to Laura's mother two years later, and she told me that Laura had remained well, and off antibiotics.

It is very interesting to me that the federal guidelines experts found no association between allergies/sensitivities and fluid in the ear. There is much in the medical literature which does indicate such an association. As a practitioner who does a great deal of allergy work, I have often seen this association with my patients. Allergy problems can affect people in many different ways, occurring in many different parts of the body. Inflammation and swelling of the eustachian tube, bronchial tubes, and sinuses are just some of the effects. When the eustachian tube swells, the fluid which accumulates in the ear cannot drain properly down the tube, creating a perfect setting for bacteria and viruses to grow. When we treat the infection with an antibiotic, we only kill the bacteria, and do not change the reason the bacteria have been able to grow there in the first place. This may very well be why the ear infections return.

In one study, 104 children who had recurrent fluid in the ear were evaluated for food allergy. Patients were evaluated with a tympanogram and through clinical evaluation. Those who were allergic to foods excluded those foods from their diet. They did not eat the foods they were allergic to for sixteen weeks. Eighty-one or 78% of the 104 children had documented food allergies.[23] When the elimination diet was utilized, the ear symptoms resolved in 86% of the patients. When the offending foods were added back into the diet, 94% had a recurrence of their allergic symptoms, including the fluid in the ear. The following is a list of the most reactive foods found among the children and the number of children that had each one:

Cow's milk (31)   Corn (12)
Wheat (27)   Orange (8)

Egg white (20)   Tomato (4)
Peanuts (16)   Chicken (4)
Soy (14)   Apple (3)

Most of the children were allergic to more than one food. The number of children having only one food allergy was 11 (13.6%), the number having 2–4 food allergies was 66 (82.5%), and the number having 5–7 food allergies was 3 (3.7%). Only one child had 8–10 food allergies. The importance of food allergies has been reported in reference to nasal congestion and runny nose as well. According to this same study, food allergies are the most common underlying causes of these two respiratory symptoms in young children.[23] Another study correlated food allergy with ear disease in 87.5% of all diseased patients.[24] This is why some diet modification may be necessary as part of The Block System for Treating Ear and Respiratory Infections. Once you understand how allergies and sensitivities affect the body, you can see how they can underlie so many different medical problems.

When an allergen enters the body through the skin, mouth, or nose, it causes many chemicals to be released. These chemicals can cause inflammation, swelling, and the release of fluids in an attempt to get rid of the allergens (*see* Chapter 3). This natural attempt to rid the body of something foreign can be beneficial when it is fighting bacteria or viruses. When it occurs because of allergies, the fluids, inflammation, and swelling can encourage the development of bacterial and viral infections.

Often a doctor is tempted to prescribe medication to cover up the symptoms. As I mentioned in Chapter 3, when you do that, it interferes with the body's ability to use its innate and acquired immune system. Chances are you will continue to have infections if you don't let your body learn how to deal with them.

Jane had been given prescriptions for antibiotics each time she had one of her frequent sinus infections. She also had many allergies. Soon after she became my patient, she called to say she had another sinus infection. I told her what she could do instead of taking an antibiotic. I explained The Block System for Treating Ear and Respiratory Infections.

Jane was apprehensive at first. She had been receiving antibiotics for so long and so frequently that she thought she depended on them. I told Jane that I could always prescribe an antibiotic later if her immune system did not handle it. She called back ten days later to say, "I did it! I got well on my own." She was very pleased to know that she could recover without antibiotics.

I expect that in the future Jane's system will respond more quickly each time she gets sick until she just doesn't get sick anymore.

In children, there appears to be a relationship between having certain antibodies to foods and the later development of different antibodies to inhalants (pollens of grasses, weeds, and trees). It has been shown that children whose parents have certain inhalant allergies have a higher susceptibility to food sensitivities. They will more often develop inhalant allergies than children with low food susceptibility. Fifty percent of the children with *high* susceptibility to food allergies developed inhalant antibodies to grass pollen, whereas only 16% of the children with *low* susceptibility acquired the inhalant allergies. Fifty percent of the "high" group but only 14% of the "low" group developed an allergy to cat dander.[25]

Some inhalants show immunological cross-reactivity with specific foods. If you are allergic to a certain inhalant, you are more likely to be allergic to certain foods, and vice versa.

Most allergists I have spoken with tell me that children under the age of three do not have allergies, and it is, therefore, useless to do allergy testing with them because they do not react to skin testing. I do not agree. These same allergists have also told me that they do not test very much or very often for foods, even with older children and adults. The allergists have told me that this is because an allergic reaction to a food is immediate. As soon as one eats the food, some adverse reaction occurs and the person knows that an allergic response has occurred. All they need to do is avoid eating the food in the future. No more problems.

However, the relationship between food reactions and inhalant reactions changes things. Evaluating someone for food allergies now becomes very important in the long-term scheme of things. If a child could be evaluated and treated for food problems before developing inhalant allergies, would we be able to prevent the inhalant allergies altogether? At present, the answer to this question is not known. It does appear this could be the case, though. I have observed in many cases that when we treat the food problems, the inhalant problems improve as well, without ever treating them directly. If this proves to be the case, then it will be extremely important to improve on the ways in which we introduce food products into a young child's diet.

This same study reported that an infant could become sensitive to foods when the pregnant mother eats some foods in excess. It suggested that breastfeeding could be used as a preventive measure against these allergies. "Breast milk offers several undisputed advantages over cow's milk, e.g., it protects against gastrointestinal and respiratory infections. The delayed introduction of solid food has been associated with a significant prevention of atopic (allergic) diseases."[25]

Breastfeeding Reduces Ear Infections

One study looked at the records of 1,013 infants who were followed during the first year of their lives. Forty-seven percent (476 infants) had at least one ear infection, and 17% (169) had recurrent ear infections. Infants who were exclusively breastfed for four or more months had half the average number of acute ear infections than did those who were not breastfed at all. The ones who were exclusively breastfed had 40% fewer acute ear infections than those infants whose diets were supplemented with other foods prior to four months. The recurrent ear infections rate in infants exclusively breastfed for six months or more was 10%. Those who were not breastfed for at least four months had twice the number of ear infections. Infants who were breastfed but also received formula supplementation prior to four months of life had approximately three-fourths the risk of acute ear infections compared with the group that were not breastfed at all.

The longer one breastfeeds and does not supplement with formula or other food, the more significant is the reduction in acute ear infections during the first year of life. The American Academy of Pediatrics recommends that exclusive breastfeeding should continue for four to six months.[26]

Breastfeeding needs to be encouraged even more than it has been. Many studies indicate that breast milk has significant protection against respiratory and gastrointestinal infections. It has also been proposed to prevent allergies. When we delay the introduction of solid foods into an infant's diet by breastfeeding, it has been shown to prevent allergies.

Smoking and Ear and Respiratory Infections

Clean, nonpolluted air is extremely important to the health of our children. We do not have to pollute the air with cigarette, cigar, or pipe smoke. We have a choice. We certainly have control over whether we light up on our own private property. I always encourage parents who smoke to quit. Minimally, I require that they never smoke or allow anyone else to smoke in the house, car, or any other shared air space with a child even if the child is not at home. Secondhand smoke is that serious.

In addition to the increased risk of cancer, heart disease, asthma, and emphysema from passive smoke, children around smoke are more likely to suffer recurring bouts of ear infections.

The negative effects can be seen even when the mother smokes during pregnancy. It was found that heavy maternal smoking was a significant risk factor for recurrent ear infections. Heavy maternal smoking increased the risk by three times for recurrent ear infections, particularly if the infant weighed less than 7.7 pounds at birth.[27]

The Smoke Screen

It may seem like an overwhelming task to rid the air you breathe of smoke with the large numbers of smokers out there and with the tobacco companies' strong new advertising campaigns. When I go out to eat at a restaurant, I only sit in nonsmoking sections, preferably with their own air system, one that does not share its air in any way with the smoking section. I have told owners and managers that I will not eat in their establishment because of the smoke in the air. I usually leave my card and tell them if they ever go completely nonsmoking, to please call me. I would like to eat there when it is smoke-free. Two restaurants have converted to totally nonsmoking since my request. And guess what? Their revenues increased! If nonsmokers do not let the establishments know how they feel, we may never have a voice in this important health issue.

Although you only have direct control over your own homes, we as consumers do have a great deal of influence outside our homes. When we speak out, we help make our communities a little safer and healthier for our children and ourselves. Protecting your children by speaking up on important health issues that affect them and cleaning up their environment is also a part of The Block System for Treating Ear and Respiratory Infections.

The best way to rid your air of smoke is to prevent smoke from getting into your air in the first place. Sometimes you may need to rid the air of existing smoke. Removing smoke from the air does not mean covering the smoke smell with a fragrance. Doing this only makes a bad situation worse. Instead of smelling the toxic smoke, you cover one smell with another smell. Removing the odor rather than covering it with another odor can leave the air cleaner and safer. (See below for some suggestions on how to do this.)

Other Controllable Toxins

There are many other pollutants that have become well established in our culture and are in our environment as a result of marketing. These substances are not necessary to our lives and, with just a few small changes, could easily be eliminated from our homes. I'm referring to fragrances. I'm not just pointing to colognes and perfumes. You can find fragrances in practically everything from hand soap, hair spray, cleaning products, laundry detergent, fabric softeners, and chlorine bleach, to lipstick, deodorant, wood polishes, floor waxes, cleaning powders, toilet cleaners, tub and tile cleaners, and dishwasher soaps.

People spray fragrances throughout their houses and cars, or plug fragrances into the electric outlets so that the heat will make them stronger. Companies add a fragrance to the return air vents so it will permeate an entire building. You can hang an air freshener in the corner or drip some fragrant oils on your lightbulbs or even light a scented candle or burn incense so fragrance can be everywhere. Then we splash on perfume.

Why are we using so many fragrances and what are we trying to cover up? Clearly this is overkill. But more important, these fragrances are not natural. They are chemicals, developed in laboratories to smell like the real thing. These substances are usually formulated from petroleum products. We don't like to breathe gasoline when we pump it into our cars, do we? We would never consider putting gasoline all over our bodies or spraying it all over our homes. But that may be what you are doing when you use these artificial products.

It is no wonder more and more people are complaining of problems with these fragrances. It is due to the overexposure of toxins. People with asthma, allergies, and sensitivities suffer the most, but none of us is immune. The overuse of these fragrances can provoke symptoms in previously healthy people. It is similar to the latex glove allergies we are currently seeing. Since medical personnel have increased their use of latex gloves, their overexposure to the substance has made a growing number of these people sensitive to it. Some have even had life-threatening reactions to the latex. The same thing is happening with fragrances. Fragrances, however, do not even have the same necessary use as latex gloves. Fragrances can be avoided if we choose.

If we want to rid our air of odors, there are many wonderful and effective tools to help us do that. There are air filters, ozone machines, charcoal and lava rocks, and plain old baking soda. We can now choose unscented cleaning products as well as personal products. There are alternatives.

For children with allergies and sensitivities, the benefits of eliminating artificial fragrances from the home environment are very important and can help improve reactions that lead to ear and respiratory infections.

I recommend that parents use unscented, nontoxic products. If you feel you must have a fragrance in the air, try cooking apples and other sweet fruits, which can put wonderfully natural fragrances in the air (if you or your child is not allergic to apple). You can also eliminate odors with baking soda, and if you or your child are not allergic to anything in the air, open windows on breezy days.

The significance of allergies and the association with illness cannot be overemphasized. It amazes me how many different medical problems might be related to allergies. I am currently participating in an FDA-supervised study on the relationship of allergies to many different medical disorders. Enzyme potentiated desensitization (EPD) is a very exciting "new" allergy treatment. It has been available in England for over thirty years and is now available in the United States, through doctors like me who are involved in the FDA study. EPD appears to be effective for ear infections, asthma, nasal symptoms, chronic cough, chronic sinusitis, general allergy symptoms, headaches, skin problems, and hives. Since most of these disorders are commonly thought to be allergy related, it is not surprising that an allergy treatment would cause improvement. However, in addition to these typical allergy symptoms, EPD has also shown promise in the treatment of disorders such as hyperactivity, attention deficit, epilepsy, depression, chronic fatigue, arthritis, and Crohn's disease. With such a diverse range of illnesses responding favorably to an allergy treatment, it makes me wonder what other problems we live with that could be related to allergies.

Chapter 8

The Intestinal Tract Is Important Too!

Give Me an Antibiotic

When I was a young mother, I thought that there was nothing wrong with giving my children antibiotics. It did not occur to me that my children might have a viral infection instead of a bacterial infection. If that were the case, the antibiotics would be worthless. I certainly did not know that there were any adverse effects to using antibiotics. I thought that if the antibiotic was appropriate, it would work, but even if it did not work, there would be no negative effect. Nothing lost, nothing gained.

My children's pediatrician had been in practice for many years and was very wise. He was not quick to prescribe antibiotics. I sometimes fell into the trap of asking for an antibiotic "just in case." I remember several times when my brother was coming to visit with his children and one of my children was sick. My pediatrician did not think my child needed an antibiotic but I asked for one anyway, because I wanted my child to be well for the visit. While the pediatrician did not think the child needed the antibiotic, he usually gave me one if I requested it.

I did not know, and the pediatrician probably did not

know, that there were reasons *not* to give antibiotics. There are side effects to antibiotics. The side effect of greatest concern is an allergic reaction to an antibiotic.

Other concerns are the ones I mentioned in Chapter 2, concerning bacterial resistance. By the 1950s, just ten years into the use of antibiotics, bacterial resistance had already occurred. Instead of realizing that we physicians might be abusing and misusing antibiotics, the drug companies just figured out a way to get around bacterial resistance. They developed newer, stronger, more broad-spectrum antibiotics to treat the bacteria which had survived and become resistant to the original antibiotics. We cannot win this contest with bacteria. The bacteria will continue to win because the bacteria will continue to develop resistance to any new drugs that we develop. We are now using stronger antibiotics for what used to be minor infections. We should learn from this lesson, and use more discrimination from this point on.

Another factor we need to concern ourselves with is the problems that antibiotics can cause in the gastrointestinal system. First of all, when an antibiotic kills off the bad bacteria in the body, it also kills off the good bacteria, particularly in the gut. There are many "good" bacteria in the gut which help us break down and digest foods properly. When we give a young child an antibiotic and kill off the "good" bacteria, we immediately risk creating problems with digestion in the future.

When my own children were young, their pediatrician would recommend that I give them Lactobacillus acidophilus whenever he prescribed an antibiotic. By giving my children this "good" bacteria, I was able to replenish the "good" bacteria and help to normalize the gut.

This practice of recommending Lactobacillus acidophilus appears to have been discontinued by most doctors. Most of the patients I see tell me that it was never recommended to their children even if the children were on long-term antibiotic treatment. Some say their doctor recommends it only if the child has diarrhea as a result of antibiotic treatment. I think that these "good" bacteria should be used anytime a child is prescribed an antibiotic. It cannot hurt and it certainly could help. Nonetheless, I have had doctors tell me that there is no reason to use the "good" bacteria replacement because nothing adverse occurs with the use of antibiotics.

I think this is a case of "If you don't look, you won't see." Before I began looking at the gut for clues, I did not know that the gut could be the source of many chronic medical problems. When I first started my practice, I began using a specialty lab to look for gut problems. I looked for and found overgrowth of yeast and pathological bacteria in a high percentage of my patients. I also found depletion of good bacteria. I did not look for parasites, so of course, I never found any. I had been taught in medical school that parasites were rare in the United States. The patients who had parasites were usually those who had done a great deal of traveling, but I heard other physicians talking about how frequently they found parasites in certain groups of patients.

I wasn't convinced at first, but began looking, and when I looked, I found. I was amazed at how many of my patients had parasites. I would say that about 25% of my patients have parasites, about 50% have some type of pathological bacteria, and about 90% have an overgrowth of yeast. Yeast, particularly candida, is normally found in the gut in small amounts. When antibiotics kill off the good bacteria, the yeast can grow even more. Many physicians do not believe this matters. They do not think that having a gut "out of balance" makes any difference to our health. This is one of those concepts that takes only a little common sense. If we take an antibiotic, it can kill off the good bacteria that help our food break down so that it can be digested. When this occurs, there is now an opportunity for other bacteria and parasites to grow. Surely this would affect our health. If 25% of my patients have parasites, does that suggest that 25% of the general population who do not feel well might also have parasites?

While the importance of replacing the good bacteria when you kill it off with antibiotics does not appear to be well accepted by physicians, it does, however, seem well accepted by patients. Before coming to The Block Center, many of my patients had decided on their own to take a replacement supplement for the "good" bacteria. Some eat yogurt to provide the replacement bacteria. One study that looked at adding yogurt to people's diets (450 grams per day for four months) showed a beneficial increase in calcium levels and also an increase in the production of certain immune system cells. The study concluded that the reason that the yogurt worked in this manner was because of the presence of the live "good" bacteria in the yogurt.[28] I usually recommend that patients take an oral nutritional supplement containing "good" bacteria. Many people, particularly those with chronic ear or respiratory infections, are often sensitive to dairy products. In those cases, and because one would have to eat a great deal of yogurt to match the study subjects, it is often easier to take the supplement. This is part of The Block System for Treating Ear and Respiratory Infections.

Chronic Health Problems and the Gut

When we cannot digest our food properly as a result of problems and imbalances in the gut, we can suffer many symptoms and illnesses. Our gut is responsible for converting all foods and nutrients into a form the body can use to function, grow, and repair itself. When this process is not working, various problems can begin to occur. Some problems in the stomach come about from what is called the "leaky gut syndrome." Leaky gut is a clinical disorder that can occur when the integrity of the stomach and intestinal tract is compromised by parasites, bacteria, or an overgrowth of yeast, and is associated with increased gut permeability. When our gut is more permeable, larger food particles can be absorbed into the body. This can lead to further food sensitivities and allergies and other gut problems.

Infants have a similar problem during their first year of life. The infant's intestinal tract is very porous at the start of life. This is why it is best to avoid feeding an infant proteins and solid foods. These foods can be absorbed through the porous intestinal tract, causing allergies. The same can happen when we are older if something causes our gut to again become porous. Bacteria, parasites, and excess yeast can increase the likelihood that this will occur. There are easy, safe medical tests which can determine if one has a leaky gut. I have found that these tests are best done by specialty labs that have particular expertise in doing these evaluations. A lab that only examines a stool sample every few weeks is less likely to spot a problem. I prefer using specialty labs because they look at hundreds of stool samples each day, and if a leaky gut is found, it can usually be treated.

Chapter 9

Nutrition and Other Treatments

You Are What You Eat

Anything we eat can affect how we think, feel, and act. The importance of nutrition in our health is often overlooked, even denied, by many physicians. This is not surprising, since many physicians never take a nutrition course, even in medical school. All physicians who went to school in the last twenty years did take a biochemistry course, though, and they should have learned about the importance of nutrition in keeping our bodies working. All of our biochemical processes need nutrients to work properly. Different vitamins and minerals are cofactors in these biochemical processes. If we do not have these nutrients available, our body will not function properly. It may not happen right away, but eventually we will begin to get sick, suffer aches and pains, or experience other medical problems. Sure, you can take a medication to help stop the symptoms, but if you don't get to the underlying cause of the problem, you will not get well and stay well. This is why I recommend supplements for all my patients.

"If you eat a balanced diet, you don't need to take vitamins and minerals." This is a common chant from physicians who have not had any training in nutrition. But if those same physicians looked back at what they learned in their biochemistry course, they might remember the importance of nutrition to our health.

Are All Foods the Same?

Studies indicate that our food sources today have a different amount of nutrients than they once did. These studies indicate that organic foods have more nutritional value than the foods we are able to purchase at grocery stores.[29] When our foods are grown with pesticides, herbicides, and antibiotics, it affects their content. Many foods are processed with additives, dyes, chemicals, and preservatives, and this also affects the quality of the food. Many have the vitamins and minerals processed right out of them. So unless we are all eating raw, organically grown foods, I believe we need nutritional supplements.

The RDA stands for "recommended daily allowance." The RDAs for vitamins and minerals are intended to prevent deficiencies which can lead to certain diseases such as scurvy and rickets, not to help us achieve optimal health. Many articles in the medical literature confirm that taking vitamins and minerals in doses that exceed the RDA can improve our health and *keep* us healthy.

The benefits of vitamin C for the common cold have been in the medical literature for years. Dr. Linus Pauling did a great deal of research on the subject. Dr. Pauling lived well into his nineties taking megadoses of vitamin C daily. An article in the *International Journal of Sports Medicine* reported a considerable reduction in the incidence of the common cold when patients took between 600 and 1000 mg of vitamin C per day.[30] Another study looked at children who were deficient in vitamin A. These children had lower amounts of certain immune system cells. After supplementing with vitamin A for five weeks, there was an increase in the immune cells. The study, reported in the November

1992 issue of *The Lancet,* revealed an association between nutritional supplementation and improved immune function. This study found that people who took supplements had fewer infections than the control group.[31]

Not Just Expensive Urine

A medical study of older patients was going on in my area. One doctor told me that all of the people who were participating in the study reported that they had been taking all kinds of vitamins and minerals. He laughed at the idea and said that all they were getting was "expensive pee." He was expressing the popular theory, "If you eat a balanced diet, you don't need additional vitamins and minerals" and if you take supplements, you will simply eliminate the vitamins and minerals through your urine.

This doctor was overlooking one thing—all of the participants in the medical study had to be "healthy" geriatric patients. It had not occurred to him that perhaps so many of these participants were healthy because they were taking vitamin and mineral supplements.

In recent months, there have been articles in the medical literature indicating that many physicians have begun taking vitamins and minerals themselves, such as vitamin E to prevent heart disease, but these same doctors are not suggesting to their patients that they should do the same. Seems like another double standard to me.

No Longer Alternative

According to a study published by the *Journal of the Board of Family Practice,* nutritional medicine is no longer considered to be "alternative medicine." More than 90% of the physicians responding to a survey considered nutrition to be legitimate medicine. Ninety-seven percent of the doctors said that they use diet and nutrition in their practices.[32]

Pacifiers

In November 1995, *Pediatrics* magazine reported that in a study of 845 children aged two to three who were attending day-care centers, 27% more ear infections occurred in children who used pacifiers. Mechanisms for this difference were speculated upon. Pacifiers which were not kept clean or not cleaned properly certainly would help spread bacteria. Also the increased saliva production of sucking can help spread bacteria from the mouth, up the eustachian tube and into the middle ear.[33]

Homeopathic Medicine

Homeopathic medicine may be a new idea to many readers. However, its central concept is similar to allergy treatment and immunization. It consists of giving someone a very small dose of something which, if given in a high dose, would cause the very symptoms being treated. For example, if a person is allergic to ragweed, an allergist might give that person a very diluted dose of ragweed in an attempt to let the body become desensitized to the allergen. Homeopathy uses a similar approach. A very diluted dose of a substance is given to help stop various symptoms. Because the dose is so diluted that it cannot be measured, many physicians think that homeopathic remedies cannot possibly work. That is why in the United States homeopathic medicine is considered "alternative" by many. In many other countries, homeopathic medicine is widely accepted and used regularly.

An interesting study was conducted on the efficacy of homeopathy in ear infections. One group of patients was treated with homeopathic remedies while the other group was given traditional treatments—antibiotics, nasal drops, antifever medications, and decongestants. Outcome was measured by improvement after three hours, duration of pain, duration of fever, the need for additional therapy, and the number of recurrences after one year.

Here are the results:

	Group A Homeopathic	Group B Traditional
Duration of pain	2 days	3 days
Duration of therapy	4 days	10 days
Percent having no recurrences after one year	70.7%	56.5%
Subjective improvement after three hours	30.2%	11.5%

Based on this study, it appears that homeopathic treatments for ear infections achieve more success than traditional treatments. This is not new information. There is information in the medical literature as early as 1880 indicating that homeopathic remedies work well for ear infections. When I'm the patient, I like to get choices, and I like to offer choices to the patient when I'm the doctor. Homeopathy is a very rational choice to offer since it has shown success even with the double-blind study standard.

Homeopathic remedies are selected by the type of symptoms one has. In this study, the following remedies were used for the following symptoms of ear infection:

Aconitum 30x globules	Sudden onset, fever, after exposure to wind
Apis mellifica 6x globules	Child likes ice on ear
Belladonna 30x globules	Inflamed red eardrum, red throat, high fever, throbbing ear pain, cold extremities
Capsicum 6x tablets	High fever, pronounced pain in ears

Chamomilla 3x globules	Ear infection after teething
Kalium bichromicum 4x tablets	Yellow nasal secretions, diffuse headache, moderate ear pain, increased temperature
Lachesis 12x globules	High, continuous fever, starts in left ear then moves to right
Lycopodium 6x tablets	Starts in right ear then moves to left
Mercurius solubilis 12x tablets	Freezing sensation, pus on tonsils, sore throat, fever
Okoubaka 3x globules	Given after unsuccessful round of antibiotics
Pulsatilla 2x globules	Fever, pronounced ear pain, given after Aconitum
Silicea 6x tablets	Mild ear pain, no fever, pus in ear[34]

And You Thought Swimming Caused Ear Infections

I think, as parents, we have all associated swimming with an increased risk of ear problems in our children. If we are talking about the outside, or external, ear canal, we would be right. "Swimmer's ear" is a common summer malady, and can be very painful, but it is not a middle ear infection; it is an external ear infection. Water from the swimming pool cannot get into the middle ear unless there is already a hole in the eardrum from a tube or perforation. It could also get into the ear through the eustachian tube, but that is unlikely. *The Journal of the American Osteopathic Association* published an article indicating that swimming may actually decrease the incidence of middle ear infections. In this study, 43% of the nonswimmers had ear infections while only 19% of the swimmers did.[35]

Xylitol Chewing Gum

Chewing gum may not be all bad. A study in the *British Medical Journal* found that xylitol chewing gum helped in the prevention of ear infections. Xylitol is a sugar from the birch tree, plums, strawberries, raspberries, and rowan berries. It has the same relative sweetness as sucrose and can be used as a sugar substitute. In addition to helping prevent ear infections, it has been shown to help prevent dental cavities. Xylitol chewing gum users showed a decrease in the number of ear infections, compared with children who chewed gum with sucrose as the sweetener. Xylitol specifically reduces the growth of the bacteria Strep pneumoniae and S. mutans. Since Strep pneumoniae is one of the most common bacteria associated with ear infections, the xylitol gum apparently reduced the bacteria in the area. Three hundred and six children participated in the study. There were 149 in the sucrose group and 157 in the xylitol group. Children chewed gum for two months. In the sucrose group 20.8% had ear infections while only 12.1% of the xylitol group had ear infections. Two children in the xylitol group had diarrhea. No other side effects were noted in either group. Each child chewed two pieces of gum five times a day after meals or snacks. The chewing lasted until there was no flavor left, or for at least five minutes. No other dietary changes were made.[36]

The number of ear infections seen in the sucrose group was 43 out of the 149. Only 22 of the 157 in the xylitol group had ear infections. The number of children with at least one episode in the sucrose group was 31 of 149, while the number in the xylitol group with at least one episode was 19 of 157. Those in the xylitol group who had episodes of ear infections had forgotten to chew their gum more often than those who did not have ear infections. There was no difference in the number of occurrences of ear infections in the sucrose group before or after the trial. The study was done in a double-blind fashion.

Though this study showed dramatic success in preventing ear infections by the use of xylitol gum, this is not a viable treatment for most children with ear infections. The summary pointed out that most ear infections occur between the ages of birth to two years. It would be unsafe to allow children at these ages to have gum. This treatment should not be used unless the child is old enough to properly chew the gum and understand what to do with it. This may not occur until age five. But if an older child is still having ear infections, it would be a good preventive measure to try.[36]

Chapter 10

The Block System for Treating Ear and Respiratory Infections

Preventive Medicine

My approach to all chronic problems is to look for and treat the underlying problem and then prevent them from recurring whenever possible. That is the goal with my protocol for treating ear and respiratory infections. In the previous chapters I have explained many of the underlying causes and how parents can deal with each of them. To prevent the problem from recurring, my protocol is based on developing and maintaining a healthy body. My system for treating ear and respiratory infections includes the Six Building Blocks. Each is designed to help your child be healthier and free of ear and respiratory infections.

Ninety Percent Resolve Without Antibiotics

Although studies indicate that children do better and get well sooner without antibiotics, parents have difficulty just doing nothing. It is hard for us to stand by and watch while our child has an infection. But if we don't look at the big picture, we will not have those drugs when our child really needs them. It would be even more difficult to stand by and watch your child become very ill, perhaps even die, because there were no longer any effective drugs left.

Fortunately, with this protocol, you do not have to sit by, do nothing, and hope that your child will get well quickly. With this protocol, there is something you can actively do to help your child get well.

It is recommended that you check with your doctor before starting.

The Block System

Block 1: Develop and Support a Strong Immune System

Summary: Allow the body to fight off infections so that it can use its innate system and develop its acquired system in order to be effective. Use antibiotics and other drugs carefully. Inappropriate use or overuse can inhibit the immune system as well as increase the serious problem of drug-resistant bacteria. Remember, most ear infections resolve on their own without antibiotics.

Block 2: Understand the Ear

Summary: Children's eustachian tubes are horizontal and do not drain as easily as an adult's, whose eustachian tubes are vertical. Therefore, it is not good to let children drink from a bottle lying down. Also, parents *can* learn to look inside the ear and understand what they see. A caring physician should help you do this. A red ear does not always mean an ear infection, and fluid in the ear does not usually need an antibiotic.

Block 3: Treat the Allergies

Summary: I find that allergies can cause fluid and irritation in the ears and respiratory system. Identify and treat the allergies. Remove the offending agents when possible. The most common inhalant allergens are dust, dust mites, molds, trees, weeds, and grass. The most common food allergens are milk, wheat, and corn.

Remove All Dairy Products: I have found that dairy products are one of the most likely culprits for promoting excess mucous, and inflammation and swelling of the eustachian tubes. For some children, continued use of dairy products will prolong an ear infection. Therefore, I recommend removing all cow's milk products from the diet. This includes milk, cheese, yogurt, ice cream, cottage cheese, and dairy-based formula. Wheat and corn are two other common allergens. If you are aware that your child has any other food sensitivities, then eliminate those foods as well. It is important to read all food labels to determine that none of the offending foods are present. Recheck labels on familiar foods periodically, as companies continue to alter their ingredients.

It has always seemed interesting to me that doctors are taught in medical school not to give infants foods that contain protein for at least the first nine months of their lives. These same doctors then recommend a cow's milk-based formula on day one. I have already covered the importance of breastfeeding instead of formula feeding whenever possible. Sometimes breastfeeding is just not possible, though. When that is the case, I recommend that the parents rotate the types of formulas given to their infant. One day soy-based, the next Neutramogen, then goat's milk, and then a hypoallergenic formula such as Good Start. (Though it has a cow's milk base, Good Start is formulated to create fewer allergy problems.) If these formulas are rotated, there is less of a chance that any single formula will be a problem. Unfortunately, some form of soy appears to be in all formulas, so if the child is sensitive to soy, there is not much one can do. Problems such as this make a strong case for breastfeeding.

Remove other toxins from your child's environment.

Things that can irritate, inflame, and swell the eustachian tubes are tobacco smoke, perfumes, colognes, and other fragrances.

Block 4: Support the Gastrointestinal System

Summary: As discussed above, antibiotics kill not only bad bacteria but also good bacteria. Our gastrointestinal tract must maintain a healthy balance of good bacteria to function properly. When one bacteria is reduced or absent, other organisms are free to grow, and the result is an overgrowth of yeast, bacteria, or parasites. This can be especially true for yeast. Yeast grows unchecked when antibiotics have killed off most of the good bacteria. This is why many people complain of stomach upset and diarrhea when taking an antibiotic. You can help replenish your child's intestinal tract by supplementing with the good bacteria, Lactobacillus acidophilus and bifidus. Be sure to get a product that is dairy-free.

Block 5: Good Nutrition

Summary: All the biochemical processes in the body depend on vitamins and minerals to function well. The American diet consists of foods containing preservatives, pesticides, hormones, antibiotics, dyes, and artificial flavorings. This can affect the quality of the foods. To obtain the level of nutrients we need for our bodies to function properly, I recommend nutritional supplements for all of my patients. Natural and organic foods are preferred.

Block 6: Osteopathic Manipulative Treatment

Summary: The next step toward preventing chronic ear and respiratory infections is to use very gentle forms of osteopathic manipulation to enhance the child's immune system, as well as to help keep the fluids draining from the head and neck so bacteria and viruses are less likely to be able to grow. This is an effective treatment I learned in medical school, but it is easy enough for you to do on your child at home. It only takes a few minutes and can be repeated every hour if needed. You need no special equipment, just a firm bed, couch, or cot. You can also use a changing table when working on an infant. The floor works well too.

How to Do OMT

This treatment should be done at least three times daily while your child has symptoms. After that, it is beneficial to continue the treatment at least once per day as a preventive measure. There are four parts to the treatment:

1. **Release of the lymphatic ducts (Figure 7).** The child should be lying on his or her back with the parent at the child's head. Locate the collarbone. This is the bone which stretches from the shoulder to just under the neck on both sides of the body. With fingers approximately halfway between the shoulders and the neck, allow fingers to "fall off" the collarbone toward the chest. There is usually a slight indentation in this area. Sometimes there is tenderness in the area when you push on the muscles there. You may feel a small bumpy area that feels something like a BB or small marble. Press gently on the tender area. If your child is old enough to cooperate, gently and slowly move one arm across his or her chest while still keeping a finger on the BB or tender area. If your child is too young to cooperate, go to the next paragraph. As you slowly move the arm across the body, the area under your finger softens or becomes less tender. When you find the position where the muscles soften or the tenderness improves, hold the arm in that position for 90 seconds. Then slowly and gently move the arm back to the usual position. Repeat with the other arm.

Figure 7
Release of Lymphatic Ducts

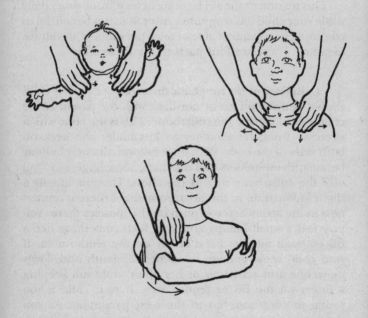

If your child is too young to cooperate with the arm moving, simply gently massage the area below the collarbone for several minutes, then proceed with the next step.

2. Effleurage of head and neck (Figure 8). With thumbs flat and pressing on the middle of child's forehead, gently but firmly, push the thumbs outward from the center of the forehead to the hairline and down the outsides of the cheeks. Do this several times. Next with the same type of pressure and using both thumbs, do the same across the nose and cheeks. Follow by doing the same thing to the neck area. Work only on one side of the neck at a time and be sure to effleurage the front and back of the neck. When doing this part of the treatment, be sure that you are always pushing the fluids toward the heart. When you are working on the face and neck, push the fluids downward.

3. Thoracic pump (Figure 9). Using the palm of one hand, push gently but firmly against the child's rib cage, stretching the muscles that lie between the ribs. Use the other hand to hold the child's arm upward and away from the body. Repeat on the other side.

4. Effleurage of the arms and legs (Figures 10 and 11). Encourage lymph flow throughout the child's body by stroking the skin on the arms and legs with an upward motion from the wrists and ankles. Use a gentle but firm, smooth, sliding motion. It is not necessary to lift your hand from your child's arm or leg until you have reached the top of the area to be treated. Always stroke toward the heart.

Repeat each of the above procedures three times daily. A video is available from The Block Center, which demonstrates these techniques on an infant and a child.

If you have any concern that your child is not getting well, or is getting worse, check with your doctor.

This treatment alone has been shown to have a dramatic effect on fluid in the ears. It works well on any type of upper respiratory infection also. If you apply these meth-

Figure 8
Effleurage of Head and Neck

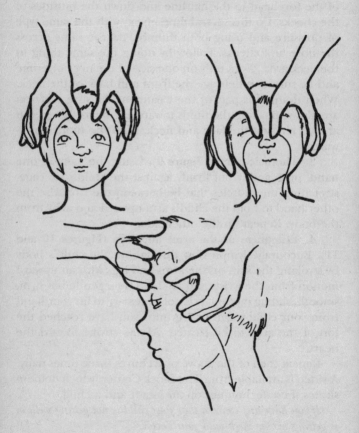

Figure 9
Thoracic Pump

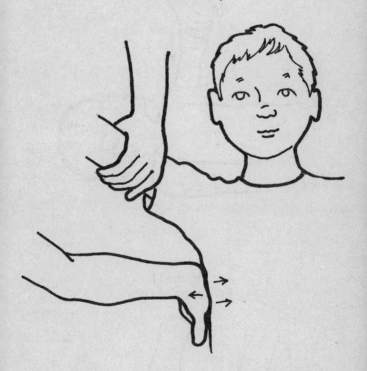

Figure 10
Effleurage of Arms

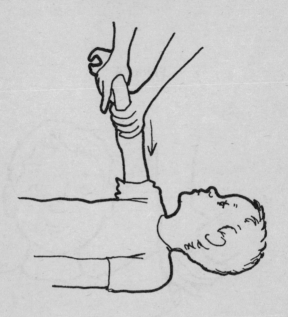

Figure 11
Effleurage of Legs

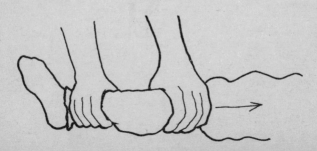

ods, along with the nutritional and other approaches discussed in this book, you can help end your child's cycle of ear infections, give him the gift of better health, and do it using no more antibiotics!

Appendix

The year 1998 saw the passing of a great man and a remarkable pediatrician, Dr. Benjamin Spock. Dr. Spock was a maverick in the field of medicine. When his book, *Baby and Child Care*, was first published in 1945, it was not readily received by his fellow physicians; in fact, they were appalled! Many thought he was crazy to advocate the things he wrote in his book, but time has proven the merits of his practical and innovative approach to child care. Millions of children in the last 50 years have grown up successfully with Dr. Benjamin Spock's wise and gentle philosophy.

Not long before his death I read an article by Dr. Spock about ear infections and antibiotics in which he expressed many of the same thoughts I have discussed in this book. Though he encouraged parents and physicians to use fewer antibiotics for ear infections, he did not have any other options for them to use in lieu of the antibiotic treatment. I was genuinely pleased that Dr. Spock held the same opinion as I did on this subject. I wish there had been time for me to tell him that I do have an effective protocol to offer parents to use instead of so many antibiotics.

It is not unusual for new ideas in medicine to meet with

a great deal of opposition when they are first introduced. I have heard it said that it takes fifty years to get a bad idea out of medicine and 100 years to get a good idea into medicine. To the benefit of our generation, Dr. Spock appeared to be ahead of the average.

Dr. Robert Mendelsohn, author of *Confessions of a Medical Heretic* and *How to Raise a Healthy Child . . . In Spite of Your Doctor,* had much to say on the subject of bad ideas in medicine. He acknowledged, with regret, that many mistakes are made in the name of good medicine. He noted the use of DES, a drug that caused vaginal cancer in the offspring of those who took it. He wrote of the outrageous uses of x-rays, such as in shoe stores so the salesperson could check the fit of the shoe. How many cases of foot or bone cancer occurred as a result of this abuse? And what happened to the salespeople who were exposed to the x-rays on a daily basis? In medicine we often get so excited about the "toys" we have available that we lose sight of our first obligation: "First do no harm." Many physicians feel that they can do whatever they wish as long as it falls under the "standard of care" in their community, even if there is harm done. Unfortunately this standard of care is often determined by the doctors who are still locked into everything they learned in medical school whether it is correct or not. (I vividly remember being taught that half of what I learned in medical school would be outdated or proved wrong by the time I graduated.)

One day when I was a medical student in the pediatric clinic, the mother of a child who had just been diagnosed with high cholesterol asked the pediatrician about the wisdom of Adelle Davis, author of several books on nutrition and health. It was obvious that the pediatrician did not know who Adelle Davis was but he did not let that stop him. He actually began yelling at the mother in front of her child, stating angrily that she could do a great deal of damage to her child if she gave her the nutritional recommendations made by Adelle Davis. I was shocked that the doctor would say these things knowing nothing of the subject. I knew who Adelle Davis was because a friend had given me one of her books when my daughter, Michelle, was sick. Of course I did not have any interest in the subject at the time; back then I still believed in the infallibility of modern medicine. But now I knew better. I wanted to take the mother aside and tell her my story, to tell her why I had gone to medical school. I wanted her to know that the pediatrician was wrong and did not know what he was talking about. But I stayed silent. To contradict the attending physician in the presence of a patient would be grounds for a failing grade. I was too intimidated to say anything.

Dr. Mendelsohn was not afraid to speak out. This brave man was ostracized by his fellow physicians because he spoke the truth. He was not as fortunate as Dr. Spock, who was finally accepted by his colleagues. Dr. Mendelsohn was still scorned by many when he died. He did leave behind many grateful patients. I had read his books long before I went to medical school; two of them helped me deal with the illness doctors caused in my daughter. It was reassuring to know that at least there was one doctor who understood what happened to us, who knew what was actually going on in medicine.

Robert Mendelsohn was warning parents about the misuse and abuse of drugs like antibiotics and Ritalin many years ago, long before I wrote my book *No More Ritalin*.

Why is medicine so slow to change? I have heard it said that we need to be cautious to protect ourselves from quacks, people who just want to take our money yet have no viable treatment. When I see the medical literature and the research that is available on the subject of antibiotics and ear and respiratory infections, I often wonder, who is actually the quack? Is it the doctor who is encouraging the patient's body to be healthy and well through natural means? Or is it the doctor who writes a prescription for an antibiotic even though everything she/he reads say she/he should do otherwise?

To my knowledge, there is no one else using the exact protocol for ear and respiratory infections that I have developed. Some use the osteopathic manipulation and others use the dietary modifications, but I know of no one else who has combined the two for this use. I know this protocol works for most people and I want everyone to have access to it. I am making it available to you now. You can decide if you want to use it or not. You can decide for yourself if it is working for you. Certainly there are times when antibiotics are necessary and even life-saving. Most of the time, however, ear and respiratory infections are not when these drugs are needed. *Using this treatment should not keep you from seeing your doctor, particularly when your child seems lethargic, is unable to eat or drink, or has a high fever.*

While my basic protocol consists of the six blocks mentioned in the previous chapter, there are other important issues that should not be overlooked while working toward good health for your child or for yourself.

I recommend that all my patients take nutritional supplements. I believe it is impossible today to obtain sufficient nutrients today exclusively from our diet. Even though I believe everyone needs nutritional supplementation, it should not prevent us from eating a good, healthful diet. Of course, just what constitutes a good, healthful diet is still under debate. But here are some important features of every healthful diet:

1. Fruits and vegetables are imperative. Unfortunately most children do not like to eat vegetables. One way to help is by setting a good example. If parents eat vegetables themselves, the children are more likely to eat them. I am not referring just to corn and green beans either. The yellow and green vegetables such as squash, broccoli and even brussels sprouts and other dark green leafy vegetables are some of the best selections. I recommend at least five servings of vegetables and fruits per day. Most children, when given a choice between the two, will opt for the fruit.

That is all right as long as they are being exposed to the vegetables some of the time.

2. Today, most children eat far too much sugar. There has been much debate about the association between sugar and behavior. I, for one, am convinced that the association exists. I have seen many children respond favorably to decreasing or eliminating sugar from their diet. In addition, sugar has been shown to have an adverse effect on the immune system and provides no beneficial nutrients, only empty calories. It should be noted that sugar can also convert into fat in the body.

We do not have to avoid sugar completely but should eat it in moderation. Complex carbohydrates, such as vegetables and whole grains, are a much better choice than sugar. Most readily available pasta and breads are processed and are no longer whole grain. Whole grain products can usually be found in health food stores as well as some grocery stores. Remember to eat fresh foods whenever possible. Avoid most packaged foods; while they may seem much easier and quicker to use, many contain dyes, additives, hydrogenated oils and sugar. After all, they are made to remain on the shelves for months. I prefer organic foods as it has been shown that organic foods have a higher level of nutrients.

3. The subject of fat is a popular one today. Everyone is trying to avoid fat. Certainly avoid deep fried foods as much as possible. But not all fat is bad; certain fats are beneficial, and avoiding those can actually be bad for you.

The worst fats are called hydrogenated fats or trans fats. They are often hidden in packaged foods and are not listed on the label. If a label says there are 6 grams of fat in a food, and lists 2 grams of saturated fat and 2 grams of polyunsaturated fat, then there are still 2 grams of fat unaccounted for. These two grams are the hydrogenated fats. These are most often found in baked goods such as doughnuts, breads and rolls. Saturated fats such as animal fat and butter, are the next worst offenders. Monounsaturated fats are usually not considered to be bad for us. Most oils are a combination of different fats but oils such as canola and olive oil are high in monounsaturated fats. Best of all the fats are the polyunsaturated fats, as they are actually considered good for us. Oils high in polyunsaturated fats include safflower, sunflower, flaxseed and grapeseed.

4. The essential fatty acids are also very important for our health and the health of our immune system. Omega 3 and Omega 6 fatty acids are polyunsaturated oils which have been shown to be very beneficial. As you can see from the list of nutritional supplements below, I always recommend some form of these to my patients. There are now many options available. I have listed evening primrose oil and flaxseed oil, but borage oil, black current seed oil and fish oils are good choices as well. One very good book on the subject of fats is *Fats That Heal, Fats That Kill* by Udo Erasmus.

Following is the list of nutritional supplements I usually recommend to my patients. Some readers may notice that it is the same list that is in my book *No More Ritalin: Treating ADHD Without Drugs*. I continue to recommend these supplements because I continue to find them effective for most individuals.

NUTRITIONAL SUGGESTIONS
(Always check with your physician before using)

Age	0–2	2–6	6–12	12 and up
B_1 (mg)	10	25	25	25
B_1 (mcg)	100	250	500	1,000
B_6 (mg)	5	10	25	50
Folate (mcg)	400	400	400	400
Calcium (mg)	200	500	500	500–1,000
Magnesium (mg)	100	150	200	100–400
Zinc (mg)	5	10	10	15
Beta carotene (IU)	5,000	10,000	25,000	25,000

NUTRITIONAL SUGGESTIONS
(Always check with your physician before using)

Age	0–2	2–6	6–12	12 and up
Vitamin C (mg)	100	200	500	1,000
Vitamin E (IU)	10	50	100	200
Evening primrose oil (mg)	500	500	500	500
Flaxseed oil (tsp)	1	1	3	3

It has already been 40 years since the medical field realized that we had a problem with bacterial resistance from antibiotic use. Will it really take us ten more years to do something about it? I fear that by then it will be too late; the bacteria may have already won. I hope it will not be 100 years before my technique for treating ear and respiratory infections finds common acceptance. As parents, you can make a difference in your children's lives and in their future. Dr. Spock taught us that. I know you will do what is best for your child. Here's to better health for all!

Bibliography

1. "Otolaryngologic Approach to the Diagnosis and Management of Otitis Media," Jung, T., and Rhee, C. K., *Otolaryngologic Clinics of North America*, Vol. 24, No. 4, pp. 931–45.

2. "Acute Otitis Media: Who Needs Posttreatment Follow-Up?," Hathaway, T.J., Katz, H., Dershewitz, R., and Marx, T., *Pediatrics*, Vol. 94, No. 2, August 1994, pp. 143–47.

3. "Otitis Media Reassessed," Shapiro, A., and Bluestone, C., *Postgraduate Medicine*, Vol. 97, No. 5, May 1995, pp. 73–81.

4. *Third Line Medicine—Modern Treatments for Persistent Symptoms*, Werbach, M., Routledge and Kegan Paul, Inc., 1986.

5. "Choosing the Right Therapy for Acute Otitis Media," English, G., *The Journal of Respiratory Diseases*, Vol. 6, No. 7, July 1985, pp. 93–100.

6. "Wise Antibiotic Use in the Age of Drug Resistance," Cohen, M., Rex, J., and Anderson, D., *Patient Care*, May 15, 1997.

7. "Abuse and Timing of Use of Antibiotics in Acute Otitis Media," Diamant, M., and Diamant, B., *Archives of Otolaryngology,* Vol. 100, September 1974, pp. 226–232.

8. "An Approach to Difficult Management Problems in Otitis Media in Children," Legler, J., *JABFP,* Vol. 4, No. 4, September–October 1991.

9. "Open Randomized Trial of Prescribing Strategies in Managing Sore Throat," Little, P., et al., *British Medical Journal,* Vol. 314, March 8, 1997, pp. 722–27.

10. "Doctors Compelled to Overuse Antibiotics," Charnow, J., *Medical Tribune,* Vol. 38, No. 16, September 18, 1997, pp. 1–7.

11. "Middle Ear Infections in Children," Brooks, A., *Science News,* Vol. 146, No. 21, November 19, 1994, pp. 332–333.

12. "Otitis and Sinusitis: Newer Drugs Boost Cost, But Usually Not Efficacy," Boschert, S., *Family Practice News,* March 15, 1994.

13. "Anti-Antibiotics," Garza, M., and Stein, S., *Chicago Tribune, Fort Worth Star Telegram,* February 2, 1996.

14. "Managing Otitis Media: A Time for Change," Paradise, J., *Pediatrics,* Vol. 96, No. 4, October 1995, pp. 712–15.

15. "The Rise of Acute Otitis Media," Eden, A., Fireman, P., and Stool, S., *Patient Care,* Vol. 29, No. 16, October 1995, pp. 22–52.

16. "The Medical Appropriateness of Tympanostomy Tubes Proposed for Children Younger Than 16 Years in the United States," Kleinman, L., Kosecoff, J., Dubois, R., and Brook, R., *Journal of the American Medical Association,* Vol. 271, No. 16, April 1994, pp. 1250–55.

17. "Treating Persisitent Glue Ear in Children," Melker, R., *British Medical Journal,* Vol. 306, January 2, 1993, pp. 5–6.

18. "Myringotomy in Acute Otitis Media," Roddy, O., Earle, R., and Haggerty, R., *Journal of the American Medical Association,* Vol. 197, No. 11, September 1966, pp. 127–31.

19. "Managing Otitis Media with Effusion in Young Children: Quick Reference Guide for Clinicians," U.S. Department of Health and Human Services, Agency for Health Care Policy and Research, July 1994, pp. 11–12.

20. "Otitis Media Panel Made 'Grievous Errors,'" Van Meter, Q., *American Academy of Pediatrics Newsletter,* 1994.

21. "The Effect of the Lymphatic Pump on the Immune Response: I. Preliminary Studies on the Antibody Response to Pneumococcal Polysaccharide Assayed by Bacterial Agglutination and Passive Hemagglutination," Measel, J., *Journal of American Osteopathic Association,* Vol. 82, No. 1, September 1982, pp. 28/59–31/62.

22. "The Osteopathic Thoracic-Lymphatic Pump: A Review of the Historical Literature," Amalfitano, D., *Journal of Osteopathic Medicine,* April–May 1987, pp. 20–24.

23. "Role of Food Allergy in Serous Otitis Media," Nsouli, T., Nsouli, M., Linde, R., et al., *Annals of Allergy,* Vol. 73, No. 3, September 1994, pp. 215–19.

24. "The Association of Otitis Media with Effusion and Allergy as Demonstrated by Intradermal Skin Testing and Eosinophil Cationic Protein Levels in Both Middle Ear Effusions and Mucosal Biopsies," Hurst, D., *Laryngoscope,* Vol. 106, 1996, pp. 1128–37.

25. "Relationship Between IgG1 and IgG4 Antibodies to Foods and the Development of IgE Antibodies to Inhalant Allergens. Increased Levels of IgG Antibodies to Foods in

Children Who Subsequently Develop IgE Antibodies to Inhalant Allergens," Calkoven, P., Aalbers, V., Koshte, P., et al., *Clinical and Experimental Allergy,* Vol. 21, 1991, pp. 99–107.

26. "Exclusive Breast-Feeding for at Least 4 Months Protects Against Otitis Media," Duncan, B., Ey, J., Holberg, C., et al., *Pediatrics,* Vol. 91, No. 5, May 1993.

27. "Passive Smoke Exposure and Otitis Media in the First Year of Life," Ey, J., Holberg, C., Aldous, M., et al., *Pediatrics,* Vol. 5, No. 5, May 1995.

28. "Influence of Long-Term Yoghurt Consumption in Young Adults," Halpern, G., Vruwink, K., Van de Water, J., et al., *International Journal of Immunotherapy,* Vol. VII, No. 4, 1991, pp. 205–10.

29. "Organic Foods vs. Super Market Foods: Elemental Levels," Smith, B., *Journal of Applied Nutrition,* Vol. 45, No. 1, 1993.

30. "Vitamin C and Common Cold Incidence: A Review of Studies with Subjects Under Heavy Physical Stress," Hemila, H., *International Journal of Sports Medicine,* Vol. 17, No. 5, 1996, pp. 379–83.

31. "Abnormal T-Cell Subset Proportions in Vitamin-A-Deficient Children," Semba, D., et al., *The Lancet,* Vol. 341, January 2, 1993, pp. 5–8.

32. "Physicians' Attitudes Toward Complementary or Alternative Medicine: A Regional Survey," Berman, B., Singh, B., Lao, L., et al., *Journal of the Board of Family Practice,* Vol. 8, Sept.–Oct. 1995, pp. 361–66.

33. "Use of Pacifiers Linked with Babies Acute Otitis Media," Niemela, M., *Pediatrics,* Vol. 96, 1995, pp. 884–88.

34. "The Homoeopathic Treatment of Otitis Media in Children—Comparisons with Conventional Treatment," Friese, K., Kruse, S., et al., *International Journal of Clinical Pharmacology and Therapeutics,* Vol. 35, No. 7, 1997, pp. 296–301.

35. "Does Swimming Decrease the Incidence of Otitis Media?," Robertson, L., Agote, M., et al., *Journal of the American Osteopathic Association,* Vol. 97, No. 3, March 1997, pp. 150–152.

36. "Xylitol Chewing Gum in Prevention of Acute Otitis Media: Double Blind Randomized Trial," Uhari, M., Kontiokari, T., *British Medical Journal,* Vol. 313, No. 7066, November 9, 1996, pp. 1180–83.

The Block System™ Health and Learning Programs

The Block System for Treating Ear and Respiratory Infections, The Video
A how-to video for parents

In this video Dr. Block demonstrates techniques which help to drain the eustachian tubes and stimulate the immune system. The easy-to-follow video includes step-by-step instructions for treating both infants and children. The techniques also work on adults with respiratory infections.

The Learn-How-To-Learn Program
This teacher-approved, doctor-designed and kid-tested interactive program was developed by Dr. Block to help children learn the way teachers teach. It is designed to help your child develop the ability to process, understand, and mentally organize information. The Learn-How-To-Learn™ program draws from proven, beneficial developmental activities and converts them for home use.

Read-with-Ease Highlighter Bookmarks™
All ages can see an immediate improvement in comfort, clarity, and comprehension.

Simply lay a colored Read-with-Ease™ Bookmark flat on the page and read through it. Try all the colors and choose the one that works best for you. Package contains five different colored bookmarks. The Read-with-Ease™ Bookmarks can mark your page, help increase reading pace, and reduce eye fatigue. Most people can see better and more clearly with less stress to read longer and more comfortably.

The Learning Stone Key Chain

How to "hold on to what you learn"

Children who have difficulties learning in school are often tactile learners—they learn best through touching. These children often need tactile stimulation to help them learn through their other senses. That's where this small, smooth stone can help. Invoking the tactile senses while trying to learn may enhance auditory and visual learning. This may also help reduce unacceptable, active behavior in the classroom.

Learning with Mozart Audiotape

Dr. Block recommends that her patients listen to the *Learning with Mozart* audiotape while studying or reading. Many parents have reported that homework time is cut in half. Parents like using the tape for their reading and work as well.

Food Power 4-Kids©
The Rotation Diet Made Easy©

The Food Power 4-Kids© program is a new method for organizing, planning, and preparing meals on a rotation diet. Rotation diet is used for children who have food allergies and sensitivities. The kit contains instructions and a magnetic board with more than 150 food magnets to help parents set up and change meals for a four-day food cycle. Written instructions and a video by Dr. Block explain the Food Power 4-Kids© program.

No More Ritalin: Treating ADHD without Drugs
A Mother's Journey—A Physician's Approach
By Dr. Mary Ann Block
This book gives the reader an in-depth overview of Dr. Block's philosophy and medical approach.

The Block Center ADHD Program
This informational video features Dr. Block as she explains the nondrug approach used at The Block Center to treat ADHD.

No More Ritalin Seminar
Audiotape of Dr. Block as she addresses a live audience at one of the well-attended workshops she conducts around the country. Dr. Block explains the problem with the ADHD diagnosis and the limits of drug therapy. She summarizes the most common causes of ADHD symptoms that she sees at her center and how she treats them. An informative tape and an excellent complement to her book *No More Ritalin*.

Block System™ products are available at health food stores and at The Block Center.

For more information, call 1-888-Dr Block or 1-817-280-9933.

Nutri-Kids™
Vitamin A to Zinc in a Kid's Drink!

This powdered drink mix contains key nutrients, essential fatty acids, fiber, important "friendly bacteria" and no sugar. Tastes great when mixed with soy milk, water or other healthy beverages!

Finally! . . .
. . . a comprehensive, good-tasting nutritional supplement for children that I could put my name on!

Dr. Mary Ann Block

Nutritional supplements are an important part of the children's health and learning program at the Block Center. I have seen in my practice how supplements can make a major difference in how children feel and act.

All the biochemical processes in the body depend on vitamins and minerals to function properly. There are many problems and concerns with the American diet because it consists of foods containing preservatives, pesticides, hormones, antibiotics, dyes, and artificial flavorings. There are so many articles in the medical literature which confirm that vitamins and minerals help keep us healthy. But the specific supplements I recommend for children at the Block Center were either hard to find, in a pill form and comprehensive, easy-to-swallow, tasty, nutritional drink for children which contains key nutrients, essential fatty acids, fiber, important "friendly bacteria" and no sugar. Now, Nutri-Kids™ Vitamin A to Zinc in a Kid's Drink is available to all children and even adults.

Nutri-Kids™ is available at healthfood stores and The Block Center.
For more information, call 1-888-Dr Block, or 817-280-9933
Or visit The Block Center web page at *www.blockcenter.com*

Publisher's Resource Guide

Bottled Water

Mountain Valley Water
1-800-643-1501
A fine, slightly alkaline water, bottled in glass

Canned Fish
High in omega-3 fatty acids and calcium

Crown Prince
1-800-255-5063

Cod Liver Oil and Fish Oils

Carlson® Laboratories
1-800-323-4141
High in EPA and DHA omega-3 fatty acids. Available in liquid form in regular and lemon flavor. Cod liver oil and regular fish oil are also available in softgels.

DHA

Martek
1-888-652-7246
DHA is an essential fatty acid necessary for life, also available in non-fish, micro-algae form. Look for product called Neuromins® DHA in softgel form.

Free Range Chicken and Turkey
Raised without antibiotics or hormones

Shelton's
1-800-541-1833 or 909-623-4361

Green Tea

Yogi Tea and Ancient Healing Formulas
1-800-359-2940 or 1-800-YOGITEA
Also available in low-caffeine formulas

Garlic Extracts

Wakunaga of America, Inc.
1-800-421-2998

Homeopathic Remedies

Enzymatic Therapy
1-800-783-2286
Exclusive distributor for Lehning
Laboratories

Hypertension Supplement

Nature's Plus
1-800-645-9500
Call for information about their
product, Pedi-Active

Nutritional Supplements

Enzymatic Therapy
1-800-783-2286

Nature's Plus
1-800-645-9500